KIRWAN'S OPERATING ROOM TECHNIQUES

An Illustrated Guide for the Surgical Assistant

Laurence Kirwan MD, FRCS
Plastic Surgeon
Diplomate, American Board of Plastic Surgery

- »» Compact easy-to-use reference.
- »» How to be an efficient surgeon and an assistant.
- »» Step-by-step instructions on instrument and hand tying.
- »» Guidance from a Plastic Surgeon with 35 plus years of experience.

Copyright © 2022 by Laurence Kirwan

Kirwan, Laurence, KIRWAN'S OPERATING ROOM TECHNIQUES An Illustrated Guide for the Surgical Assistant. Kindle Edition All rights reserved. Duplication, distribution, or database storage of any part of this work is prohibited without prior written approval from the publisher.

ISBN

PREFACE

This book is aimed for those working in the Operating Room: surgical assistants, scrub techs, medical students, and surgical residents. I teach Physician Assistants in a Surgical Fellowship Program at Norwalk Hospital in Connecticut (sponsored by Yale New Haven Medical System). This manual teaches basic skills and essential operating room knowledge that I have learned over my career as a Plastic Surgeon for the last 35 years. I hope to lower the learning curve and increase the knowledge base for those beginning a career in the operating room or for those simply wanting to improve their surgical skills, whether it be in the Emergency Room or in Private Practice.

"If you aim for less than perfection, you will hit it every time."

Frederick J. McCoy, M.D., Dr. Kirwan's Chief at University of Missouri, Kansas City.

AUTHOR'S NOTE

For the sake of brevity, I have referred to the dominant hand as the *right* hand and the non-dominant hand as the *left* hand. If you are left-handed, please reverse *right* and *left* in the text.

Illustrations may be repeated to avoid having to flip pages.

Take a moment to become familiar with the terms wrist *pronation* and *supination*, and wrist and finger *flexion* and *extension*. If you stand with your elbows at your sides, flexed to ninety degrees and palms facing each other, rotating your palms to the floor is called *pronation* and rotating your palms upwards to the ceiling is *supination*. If you stand in the *anatomical position* with your elbows straight, palms facing forwards, the wrists and fingers are extended (straightened) when moved posteriorly and are flexed when bending the wrists forwards and when curling the fingers into the palm. It is important to understand these terms when discussing knot tying and knot cutting,

CONTENTS

1. POWER WORDS — 1
2. SUTURES & NEEDLES — 5
    Suture types — 6
    Notes on sutures — 7
    Different needle types — 10
3. GOWNING, SURGICAL GLOVES, AND OPERATING ROOM DO'S & DON'T'S — 13
4. INSTRUMENTS — 17
    Choice of needle holder — 19
    General comments — 20
    Instrument parts — 21
        A. Holding a ringed instrument — 25
        B. Holding a spring instrument e.g., forceps — 35
        C. Holding a handled instrument e.g., mallet — 36
5. PLACING SUTURES & KNOT TYING — 37
    A. Placing sutures — 38
    B. Hand tremor - how to reduce it — 51
    C. Knot tying — 53
6. SUTURE CUTTING — 91
    How to cut a suture using a straight Mayo scissor — 94
7. CLOSING WITH STERISTRIPS — 99
8. PASSING INSTRUMENTS — 105
    A. Passing a ring-handled instrument — 107
    B. Holding and passing a knife — 110

    C. Holding and passing a forceps   112
    D. Passing a closed-handled instrument   114

9. WOUND SPONGING   117

10. ERGONOMICS   119
    Tips for maximum efficiency   120

11. SAFETY   125
    Safety tips   126

12. ANTICIPATION   129

13. PRACTICE, PRACTICE, PRACTICE   131
    Practice tips   132

ABOUT THE AUTHOR   135

POWER WORDS

01

KIRWAN'S OPERATION ROOM TECHNIQUES

POWER words are words to **avoid** when operating on awake or sedated patients. **AVOID** these words!! If patients hear them, it can make them unduly anxious or, even worse, lead to medico-legal repercussions. Never joke about a patient's personal attributes. Keep conversation professional and focused on surgery, at all times. These are good rules to follow even when patient is under general anesthesia.

Power words to avoid	Say instead	Say instead
Knife	Number 15	Number 10
#15 or #10 Blade	Number 15	Number 10
Needle	25 long or short	30 long or short
Oops!	No alternative	Just don't say it!
Ambiguous words to avoid:		
OK / uh-huh		Yes
uh-uh		No
Do not joke or talk about anything that is not related to the surgery. The same applies to the scrub nurse and circulating staff.		
If you don't understand an instruction, ask for it to be repeated.		
Spell out numbers to avoid confusion.		
If you have a concern, vocalize it.		

Table 1.
Power words.

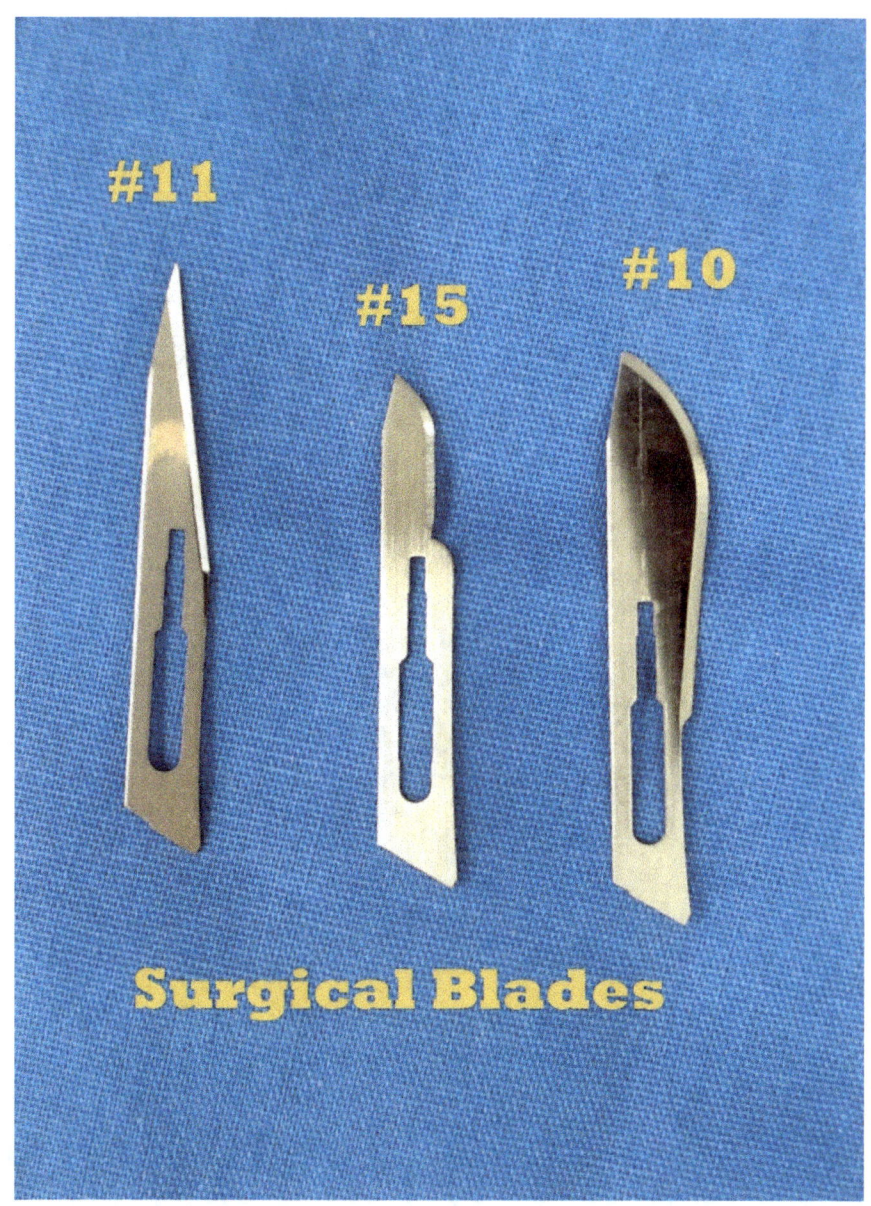

Figure 1.
Common surgical blades: #11, #15, #10.

SUTURES & NEEDLES

02

Suture types

Suture types: (learn about them and recognize them)

Absorbable		Non-Absorbable	
Braided	Monofilament	Braided	Monofilament
Vicryl Vicryl Rapide	Monocryl Fast Absorbing Plain Gut Chromic Gut	Ethibond Silk	Ethilon Prolene

Table 2.
Suture types.

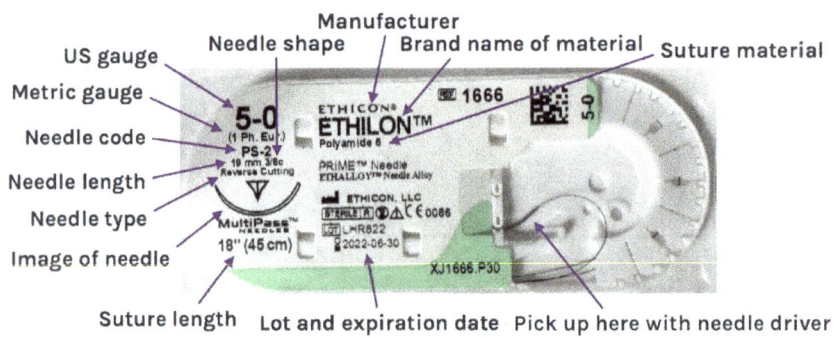

Figure 2.
Suture packet with explanatory notations. (From https://rajnursing.blogspot.com/2019/09/suture-materials.html)

Notes on sutures

>>> Prolene has a low coefficient of friction and is 'wiggly'!

>>> Nylon has a higher coefficient of friction and is also wiggly.

>>> 'Pull' out Prolene and Nylon to straighten and eliminate the springiness.

>>> With Prolene and Nylon, running or subcuticular sutures: the assistant holds the end of the suture or rests a finger on top or applies a hemostat to the non-working end to keep the end of the suture from springing up into the field, and to prevent the surgeon from accidentally pulling the stitch through.

>>> Nylon has a higher coefficient of friction than Prolene. This means that it will not 'run' and will not pull through the wound as easily. Prolene is therefore the ideal suture for a subcuticular suture since it is easier to remove.

>>> **Silk has the ideal suture tying characteristics.** The knot ties down flat and the suture does not wiggle. Silk also feels soft, unlike Prolene and Nylon.

>>> You should always use a silk suture in the red vermilion of the lip. Nylon or Prolene stick up and the sharp cut ends will irritate.

>>> For the same reason as above, use a soft absorbable suture inside the mouth such as Catgut or Vicryl.

>>> **Deep interrupted sutures.** The knot is **upside-down**. This means that the first throw is counterclockwise and then subsequent throws are reversed, as in a skin suture.

>>> Skin sutures can leave stitch marks or crosshatches across the scar. This is avoidable and should never occur. There are two ways to avoid cross hatches. The first and most common way is to perform a subcuticular suture. The second is to

remove the sutures before they bite into the tissue on either side of the incision, causing permanent scarring.

⫸ The number of days before removing an interrupted suture depends on the location. Columella and nasal tip sutures should be removed 48 to 72 hours after surgery. Other facial sutures should be removed no later than 5 days. Body and extremity sutures should be removed at 7 days. Sutures in skin that have a lot of oily sebaceous or sweat glands tend to get infected if they are not removed in the first 2-3 days.

⫸ The exceptions to the above are 5-0 and 6-0 Fast-Absorbing Plain Catgut and Vicryl Rapide. These materials cause minimal tissue reaction and in practice can be allowed to dissolve spontaneously. However, I would still recommend that they are removed according to the timelines for other types of sutures. Stainless steel staples are relatively non-reactive. Staples, however, will also leave crosshatches, except in hair bearing scalp. They can be left in for 8 to 10 days in the hair bearing scalp without any untoward effect. A common practice is to remove alternate sutures and staples at the half-way mark.

SURTURES & NEEDLES

Trade Name / Generic Name	Strength duration (days) / Absorb time (days)
Fast Absorbing Plain Catgut	• **5-7 (1week)** • (Absorb: 14-28 days)
Plain Catgut	• Up to **10 (1 week)** • (Absorb: 70)
Vicryl Rapide / **Polyglactin 910**	• **5-14 (1-2 weeks)** • (Absorb: 42-56)
Chromic Catgut	• **10-14 (2 weeks)** • (Absorb: 56-72)
Vicryl / Polyglactin 910	• **21-28 (3-4 weeks)** • (Absorb: 55-70)
Monocryl / Poliglecaprone 25	• **14-21 (3 weeks)** • (Absorb: 90-120)
PDS / Plydioxanone	• **55-65 (8-9 weeks)** • (Absorb: 180-200)

Table 3.
Absorbable sutures: strength durations & absorption rates.

Different needle types

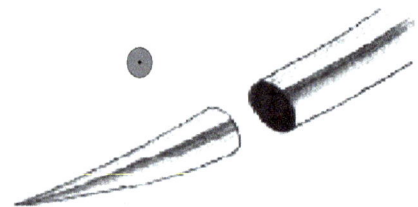

Taper. Round body with a sharp tip.

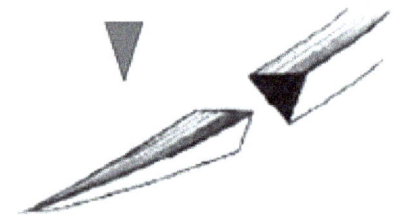

Reverse Cutting
Triangular body with sharp tip and cutting edge on the back side of needle.

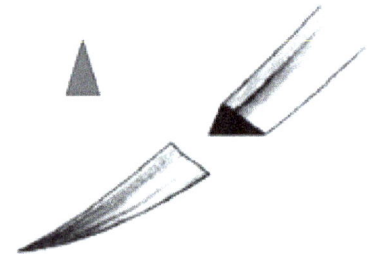

Conventional cutting
Triangular body with sharp tip and cutting edge on the front side of needle.

Figure 3a.
Common needle points and cutting edges (from https://rajnursing.blogspot.com/2019/09/suture-materials.html)

SURTURES & NEEDLES

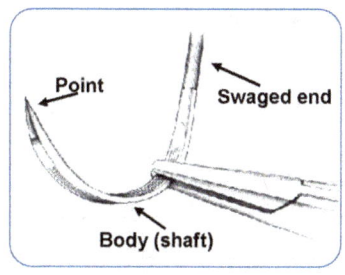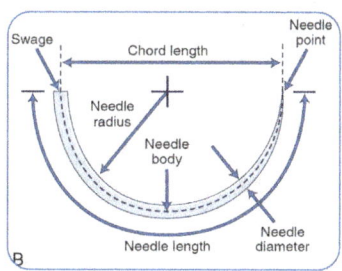

Figure 3b.
Parts of needle (from https://rajnursing.blogspot.com/2019/09/suture-materials.html)

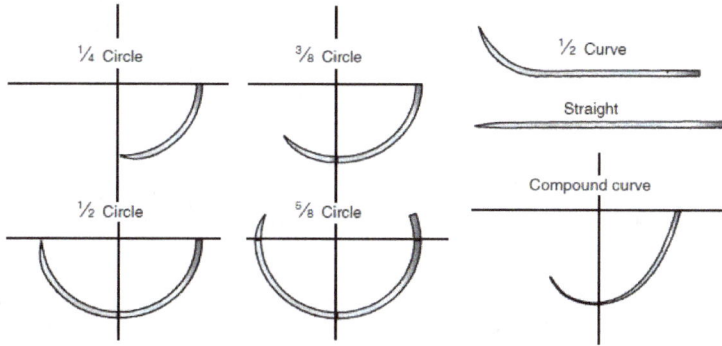

Figure 3c.
Types of needles. (From https://rajnursing.blogspot.com/2019/09/suture-materials.html)

Needle type	Examples	Point /Body
½ circle	CT	taper point / round body
	SH	taper point / round body
3/8 circle	FS	reverse cutting
	P-3	reverse cutting
	P-1	reverse cutting
Straight	KS	conventional cutting

Table 4.
Three common needle types.

KIRWAN'S OPERATION ROOM TECHNIQUES

Needle	Needle type	Needle size	Needle Type	Tissue
P-1	3/8 circle	11mm	Reverse cutting	Skin, fascia, ligament oral mucosa
P-3	3/8 circle	13mm	Reverse cutting	Skin, fascia, ligament oral mucosa
PS-3	3/8 circle	16mm	Reverse cutting	Skin, fascia, ligament oral mucosa
PS-2	3/8 circle	19mm	Reverse cutting	Skin, fascia, ligament oral mucosa
PS-1	3/8 circle	24mm	Reverse cutting	Skin, fascia, ligament oral mucosa
FS-1	3/8 circle	24 mm	Reverse cutting	Skin, fascia, ligament oral mucosa
FS-2	3/8 circle	19 mm	Reverse cutting	Skin, fascia, ligament oral mucosa
SH-1	1/2 circle	22MM	Round bodied (taper point)	Subcutaneous fat, aponeurosis, muscle
SH	1/2 circle	26mm	Round bodied (taper point)	Subcutaneous fat, aponeurosis, muscle
CT-1	1/2 circle	36mm	Round bodied (taper point)	Subcutaneous fat, aponeurosis, muscle
CT-2	1/2 circle	26mm	Round bodied (taper point)	Subcutaneous fat, aponeurosis, muscle
CTX	1/2 circle	48mm	Round bodied (taper point) **Extra Large**	Subcutaneous fat, aponeurosis, muscle

Table 5.
Needles types and tissues in which they are used.

GOWNING, SURGICAL GLOVES, AND OPERATING ROOM DO'S & DON'T'S

03

- ⟫ The Scrub Tech will usually open the surgical gown for you to insert your arms. Put both arms into the sleeves and let the Scrub pull the sleeves down so that your hands can come out of the ends.
- ⟫ Sometimes you will need to don your own gown on by picking it up off the back table, unfolding it and putting your arms into the sleeves. The Circulator or the Scrub will pull the sleeves down so that your hands come through the ends. After the Circulator has tied the back ties of the gown, hold the tab card out for the Circulator or the Scrub to grasp. Turn around in a clockwise direction so that you can grasp the waist tie again, removing it from the tab which the Circulator or Scrub will detach. Tie the long end to the short end at the front of the gown.
- ⟫ Make sure that you know your glove size.
- ⟫ Learn how to don surgical gloves by yourself. Grasp the outside (inside surface) of the cuff to don the first glove and then put your gloved fingers inside the fold of the second cuff to don the second glove
- ⟫ Learn how to don surgical gloves with a Scrub. Put one hand in the first glove and then hold the cuff of the second glove with the first gloved hand placing your other hand in the second glove.
- ⟫ If you double glove, you can put the larger size on first or second, depending on your preference.
- ⟫ If gloves are too tight, they will make your hands cramp.
- ⟫ Learn how to remove a punctured or contaminated glove. Pull the glove off over the fingers so that the Circulator can grasp and remove the glove. Repeat with the second glove grasping the cuff with your bare hand and again pulling down onto the

GOWNING, SURGICAL GLOVES, AND OPERATING ROOM DO'S & DON'T'S

fingers. Alternatively, the Circulator will grasp the cuff and pull the glove off.

》》》 Remember that everything with a blue drape is sterile.

》》》 Don't touch anything that is not sterile. If you do, then you will have to re-glove and even re-gown which is time wasting and wasteful of resources.

》》》 Keep your gloved hands between your waist and your chest. Do not hold them up in the air like an actor!

》》》 Resting the hands on the patient avoids contaminating them.

》》》 When draping the patient, do not pull drapes fully up and down. Let the drapes drop. The anesthesiologist will pick up the drapes at the top end and the circulator will pull the drapes down at the bottom. Otherwise, you will risk contaminating yourself when you pull the drapes up or down.

》》》 If you are looking for something to do, put the sterile light handles on the overhead lights. Check that the light handles are sterile before touching them.

》》》 It is a good idea to spend time with the Scrub, learning basic Operating Room techniques such as how to gown and glove. You can also acquaint yourself with names of instruments and with how the Scrub organizes the Back Table and the Mayo Stand.

》》》 Remember that that your mask is intended to cover your mouth and your nose. The nose should not be above the mask like a snorkel.

》》》 Surgical hats should cover your hair.

》》》 Wear scrubs that are provided by the facility. Do not use outside scrubs and do not go outside the surgical area without removing the scrubs.

KIRWAN'S OPERATION ROOM TECHNIQUES

- ⟫ Wear comfortable shoes or clogs that can be wiped down and/or thrown in the washing machine.
- ⟫ Nails must be short and clean.
- ⟫ Long hair should be tied up.
- ⟫ No rings or hand jewelry. No earrings that could fall into the wound.
- ⟫ If you have a beard, make sure it is enclosed in headgear.
- ⟫ If you sneeze, step back from the operating table. Do not turn your head sideways because this will render the mask ineffective.
- ⟫ If you feel faint, say so, long before you keel over.

Instruments

04

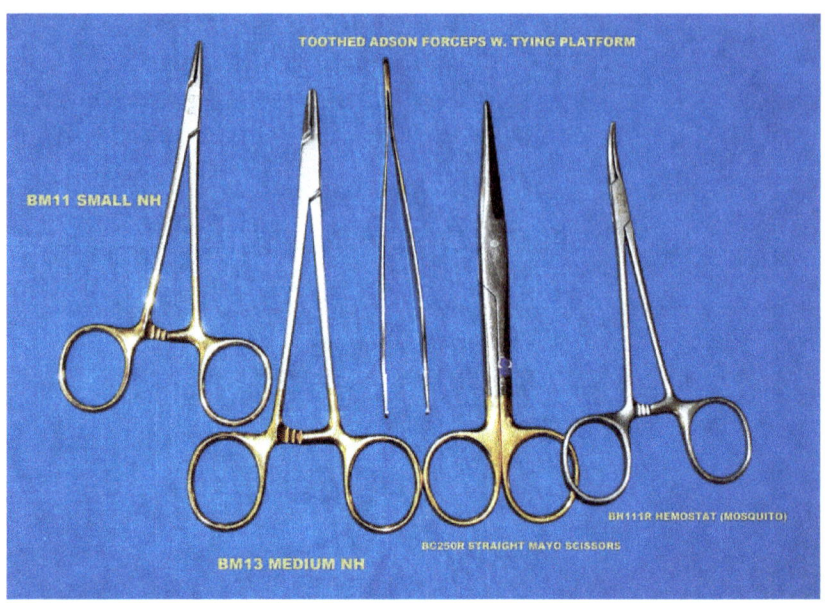

Figure 4.
A set of basic surgical instruments. Small and medium needle holders, Adson toothed forceps with tying platform, straight Mayo scissors, and a hemostat.

Needle Holder for 3-0 suture 7"(not shown)	BM066R	Aesculap
Needle Holder	BM011R	Aesculap
Needle Holder	BM013R	Aesculap
Toothed Adson Forceps	BD511R	Aesculap
Straight Mayo Scissors 5 ½"	BC250R	Aesculap
Hemostat (Mosquito)	BH111R	Aesculap

Table 6
Surgical Instruments.

Choice of needle holder

The choice of needle holder, and to some extent forceps, depends primarily on the size of the suture needle and to a lesser extent the gauge of the needle. Smaller gauge sutures generally come on smaller and thinner needles therefore requiring smaller finer needle-holders and vice versa.

Size	Needle Holder Size	Needle Size examples	Suture Size
Small	**Aesculap BM11** Converse Fine 5"	P3 P1	5-0 6-0
Medium	**Aesculap BM13** Crile Wood Fine 6:"	PS2 CPS3	3-0 4-0
Large	**Aesculap BM66 & BM67:**	PS1 FS-1 SH CT-1	2-0 3-0

Table 7.
Choice of needle holder.

KIRWAN'S OPERATION ROOM TECHNIQUES

General comments

>>> Right-handed needle holders and scissors are designed for right-handed surgeons. On a right-handed instrument the thumb **pushes** one ring, and the middle and ring fingers **pull** on the opposite ring. For a left-handed surgeon using a right-handed instrument, you must **pull** with the thumb on one ring and **push** with the fingers on the opposite ring. Alternatively, the left-handed surgeon can use a needle holder or scissor specifically designed for the left hand.

>>> A suture needle is "loaded" into the needle holder when it is placed between its jaws. The needle and needle holder combination are referred to as a **"loaded needle holder."**

>>> **NEVER** hold a ringed instrument with your thumb and index finger. Always thumb and ring finger.

>>> **Do not use hemostats to remove staples!** They are too delicate, and it will damage the hinge mechanism. Use a medium needle holder (BM13 Aesculap) or a staple remover to remove staples.

>>> **Release** a ringed instrument with a ratchet, by pressing "**up**" with your thumb whilst stabilizing or pulling the other ring of the instrument handle with ring your and middle fingers.

Instrument parts

Needle holder

A ringed needle holder (as opposed to non-ringed microsurgical and ophthalmic needle holders) and an artery clamp such as a mosquito are composed of five working parts:

1. tips (with grasping jaws)
2. square hinge
3. shank or stem
4. ratchet
5. rings

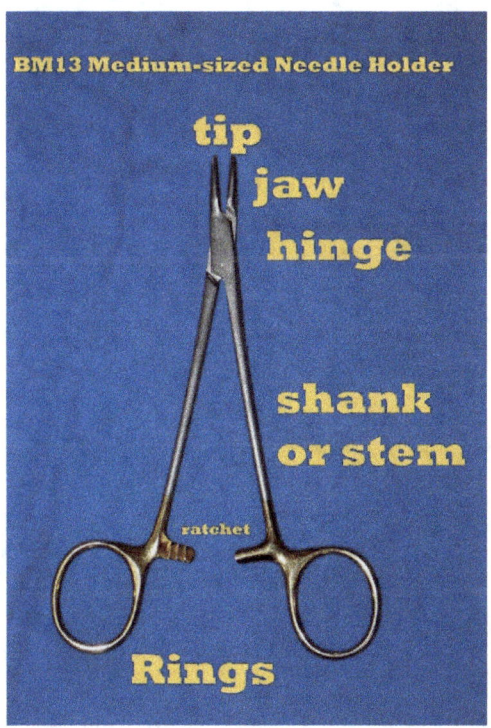

Figure 5.
Needle Holder.

Scissors

Ringed scissors such as the straight Mayo scissors illustrated in Figure 6 consist of four working parts. There is no ratchet.

1. tips (with cutting edges on the blades)
2. flat hinge
3. shank or stem
4. rings

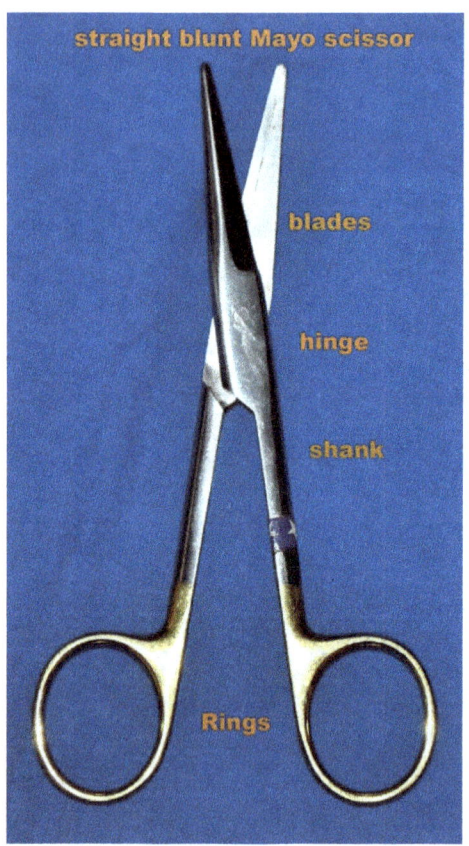

Figure 6.
Straight Mayo Scissor. The four main parts are the blades, hinge, shank, and rings. There is no ratchet.

INSTRUMENTS

Toothed Adson forceps with tying platform

Forceps such as the toothed Adson forceps with a tying platform consist of four working parts. There is no ratchet. Some forceps do have locking ratchets.

1. tips with one tooth interdigitating with two opposing teeth
2. raised tying platforms with serrated gripping surfaces
3. Ridged wider parts of the handle for gripping
4. Fused base of the forceps with bowing of each limb to provide a spring action to open the teeth when closing pressure is released

The tying platform is a flat raised platform with a gripping surface just above the teeth on each side. The tying platform is essential to grasp the needle body or shaft as it exits from the tissue. Without a tying platform, it is difficult to grasp the body of the needle so that the needle holder can grasp it.

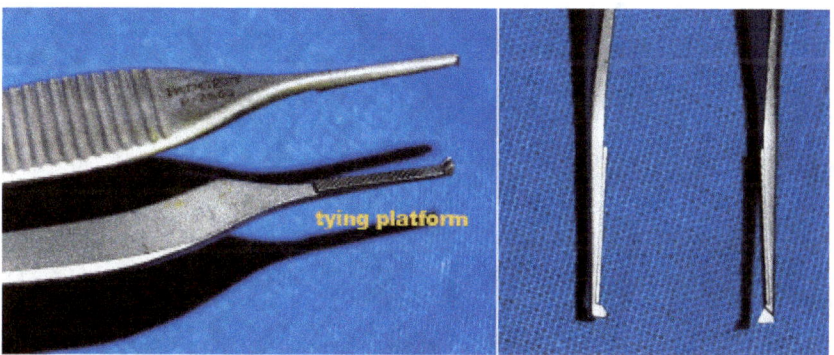

Figure 7.
Left: serrated surface of tying platform to help grip the body of the suture needle. Right: raised tying platform on each side, above the tips.

23

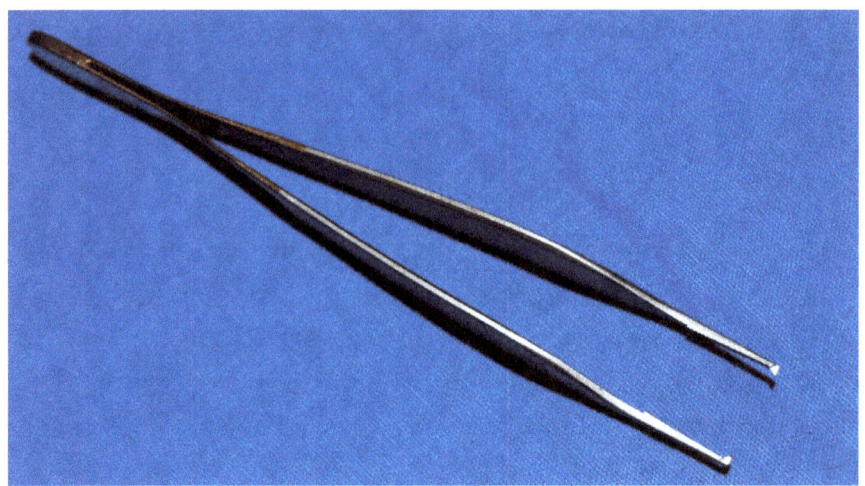

Figure 8.
Fine-toothed Adson forceps with tying platform and bowed limbs at base.

INSTRUMENTS

A. Holding a ringed instrument.

i. Tripod grip and correct positioning of a suture needle in the needle holder

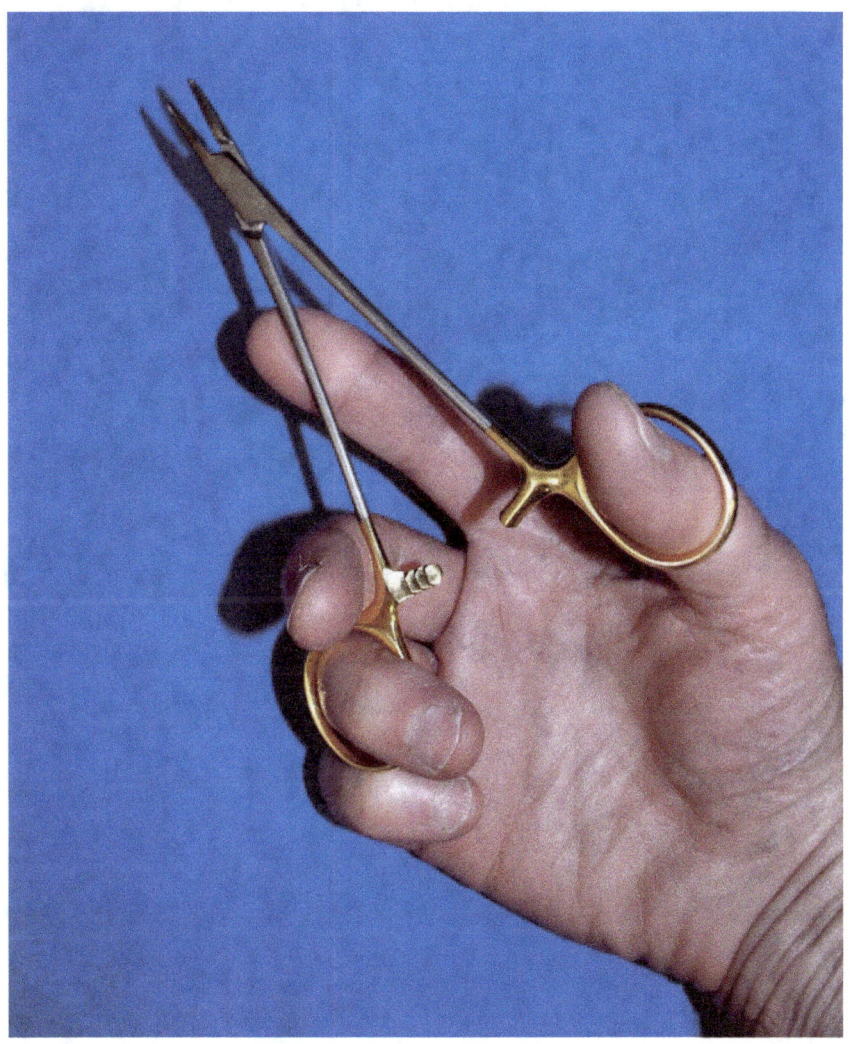

Figure 9.
Classic tripod grip shown holding a needle holder, palm view.

Thumb obliquely, halfway in one ring as shown. The index finger rests along the shank of instrument for stability and guidance. Middle finger at base of shank. Ring finger in second ring.

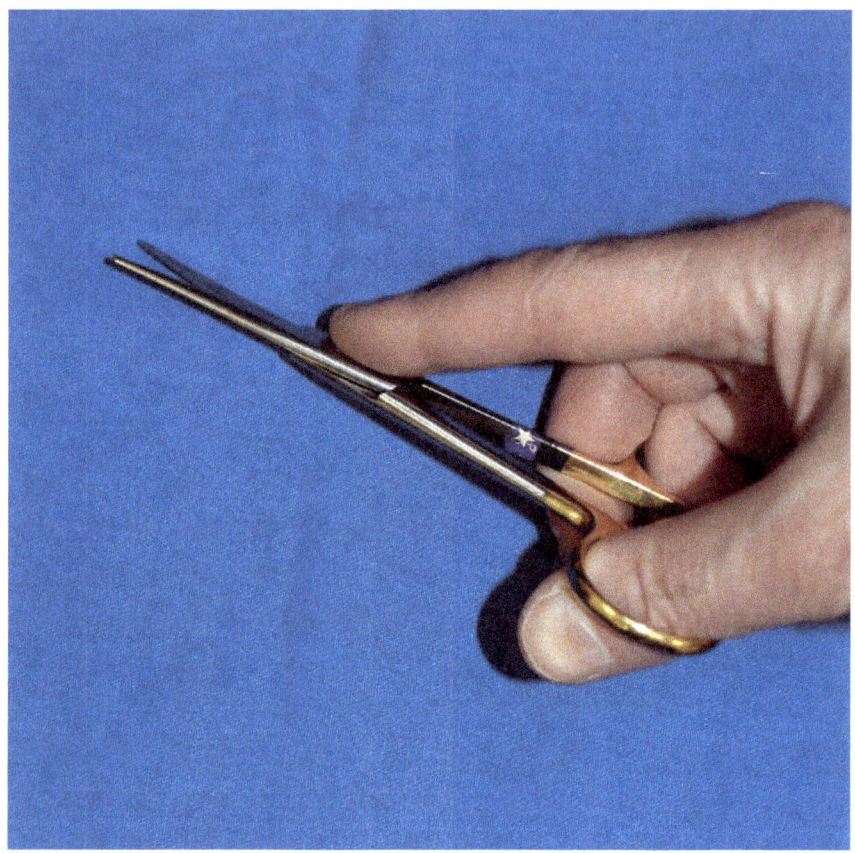

Figure 10.
Classic tripod grip holding a scissor, side view.

INSTRUMENTS

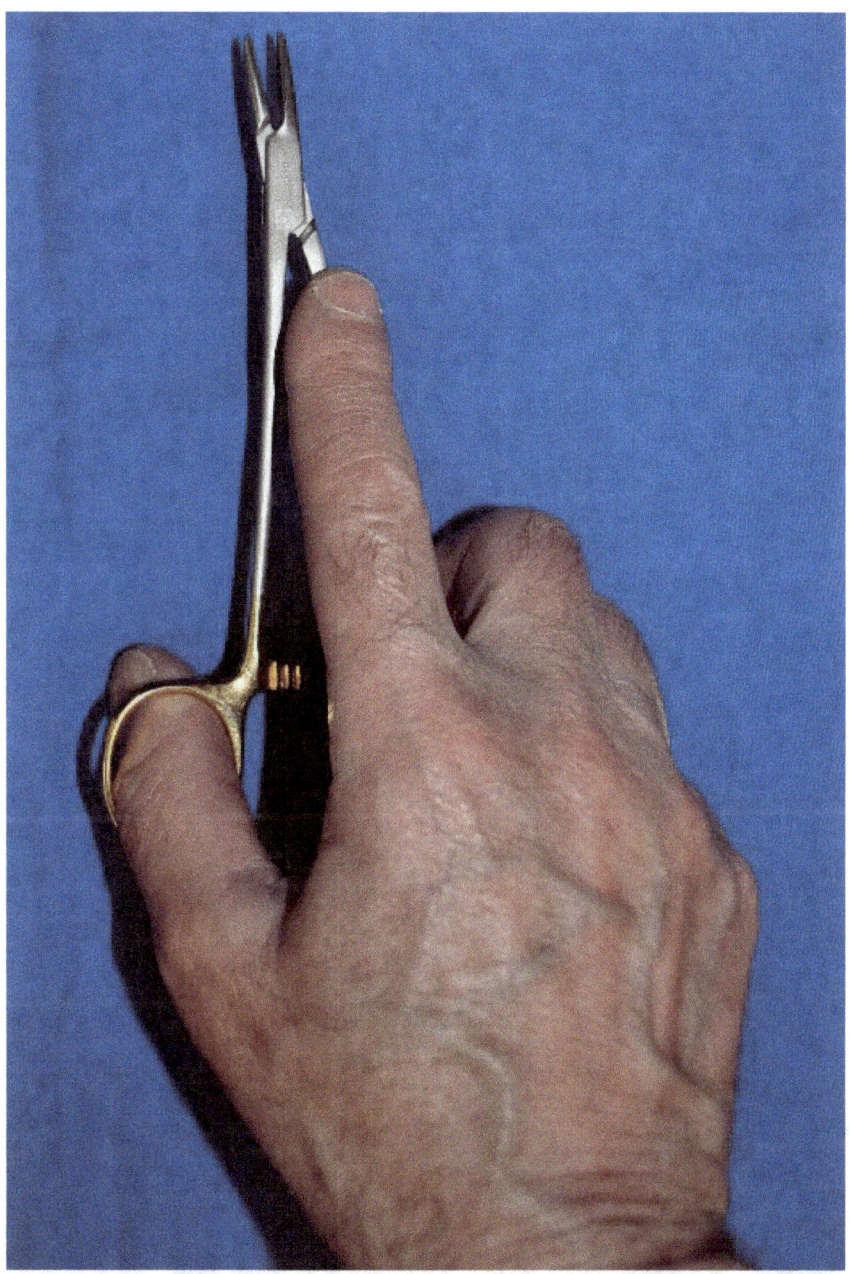

Figure 11.
Classic tripod grip holding a needle holder, top view. Index finger is straight and lies on shank, steadying (reducing shake) and guiding tip.

KIRWAN'S OPERATION ROOM TECHNIQUES

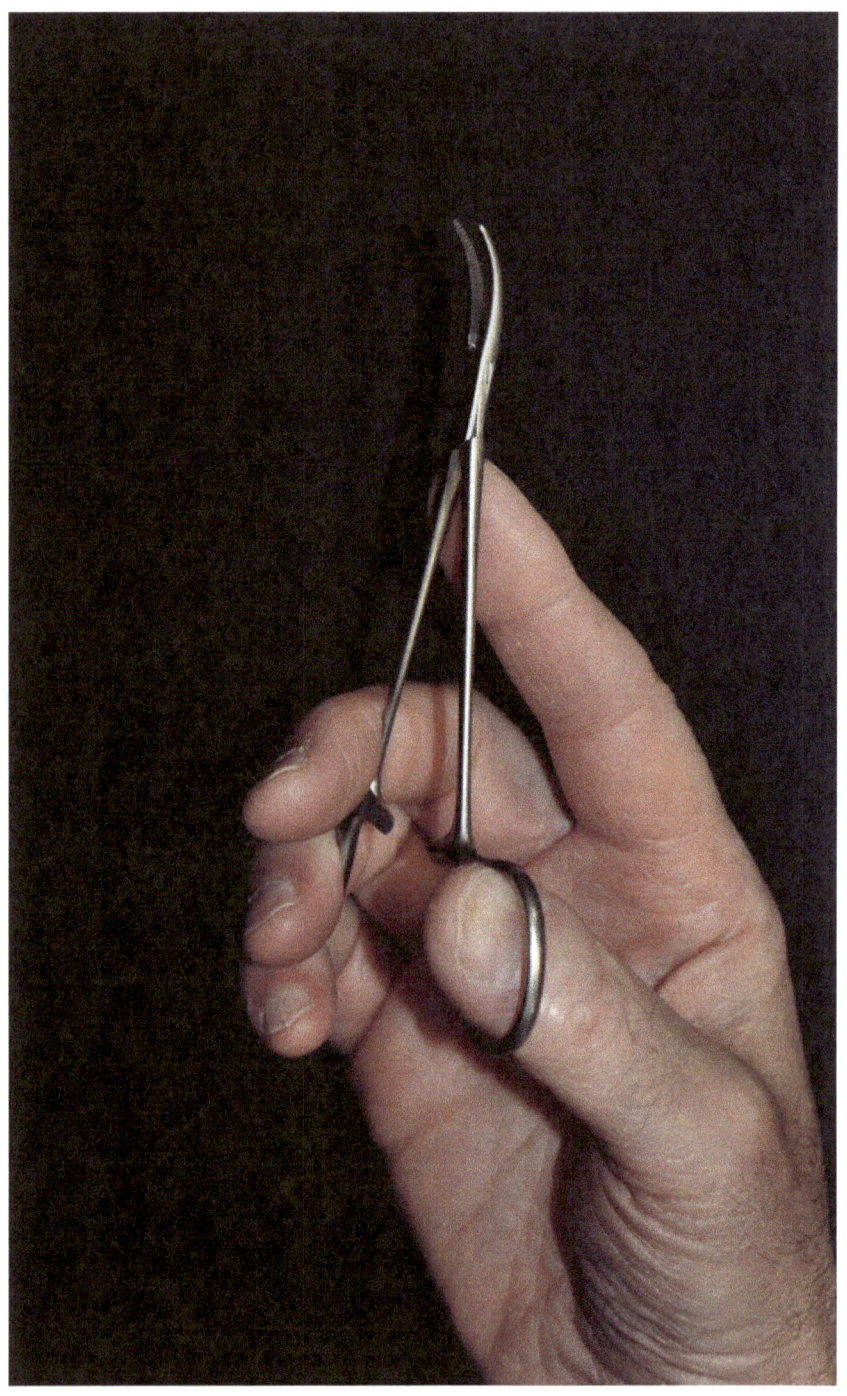

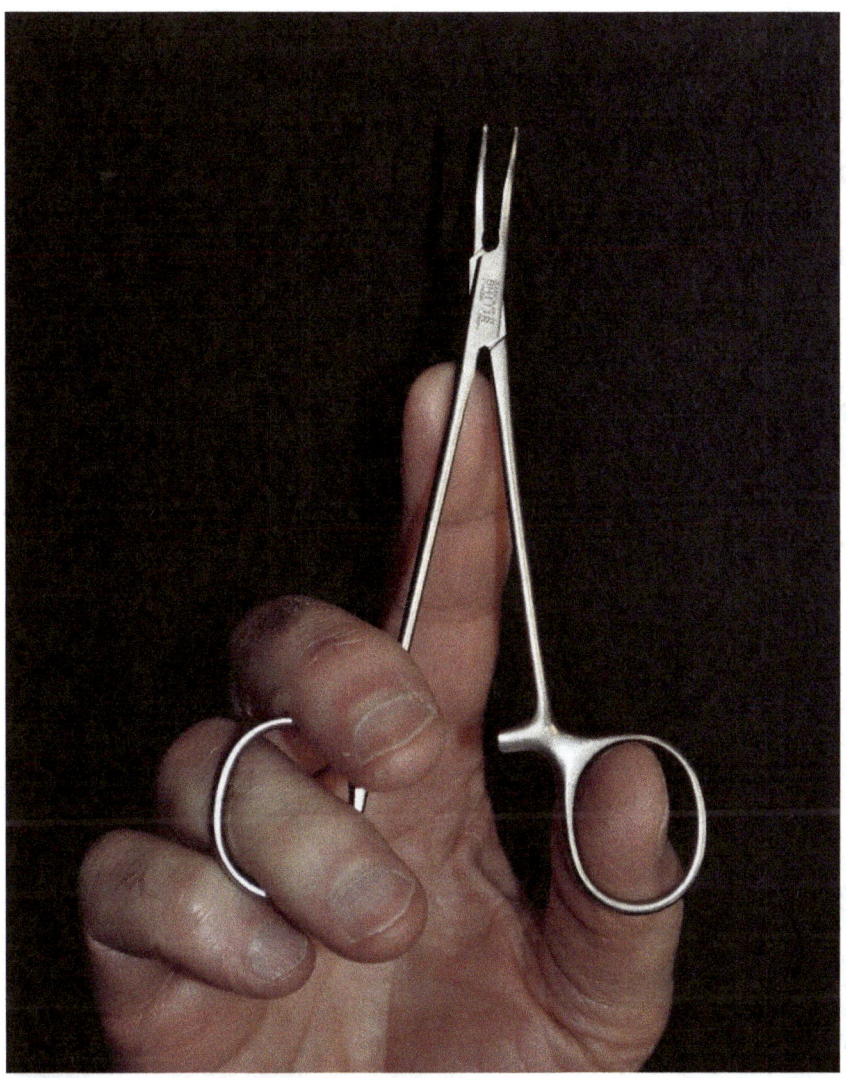

Figure 12.
Tripod grip of hemostat. Left: side view. Right: palm view.

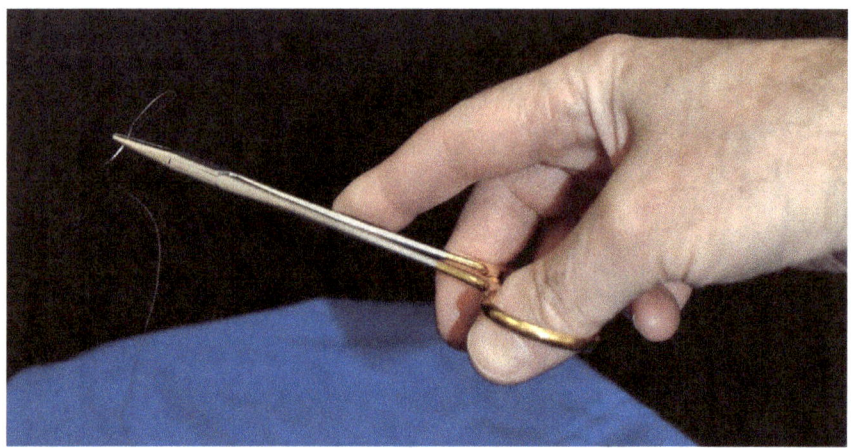

Figure 13.
The illustration above shows the correct positioning of the suture needle in the jaws of the needle holder. The needle points forward, with the needle point facing away from the index finger. The Scrub Tech may incorrectly pass the loaded needle holder upside down so that the needle faces backwards. You will then have to rotate the needle holder to the correct orientation. If you are using a needle "backhanded" as in to stitch away from you, then the needle should be reversed so that it points away instead of towards you. If you are left-handed, then the needle is reversed and placed in the "backhanded" position.

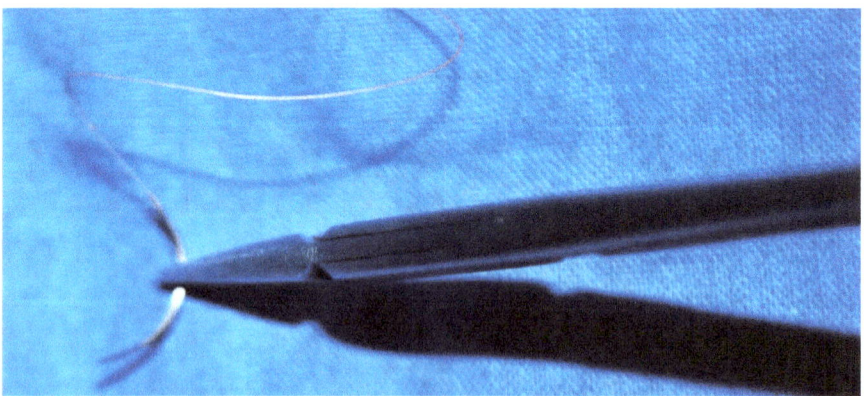

Figure 14.
Correct positioning of the suture needle loaded into the jaws of the needle holder, close-up view.

INSTRUMENTS

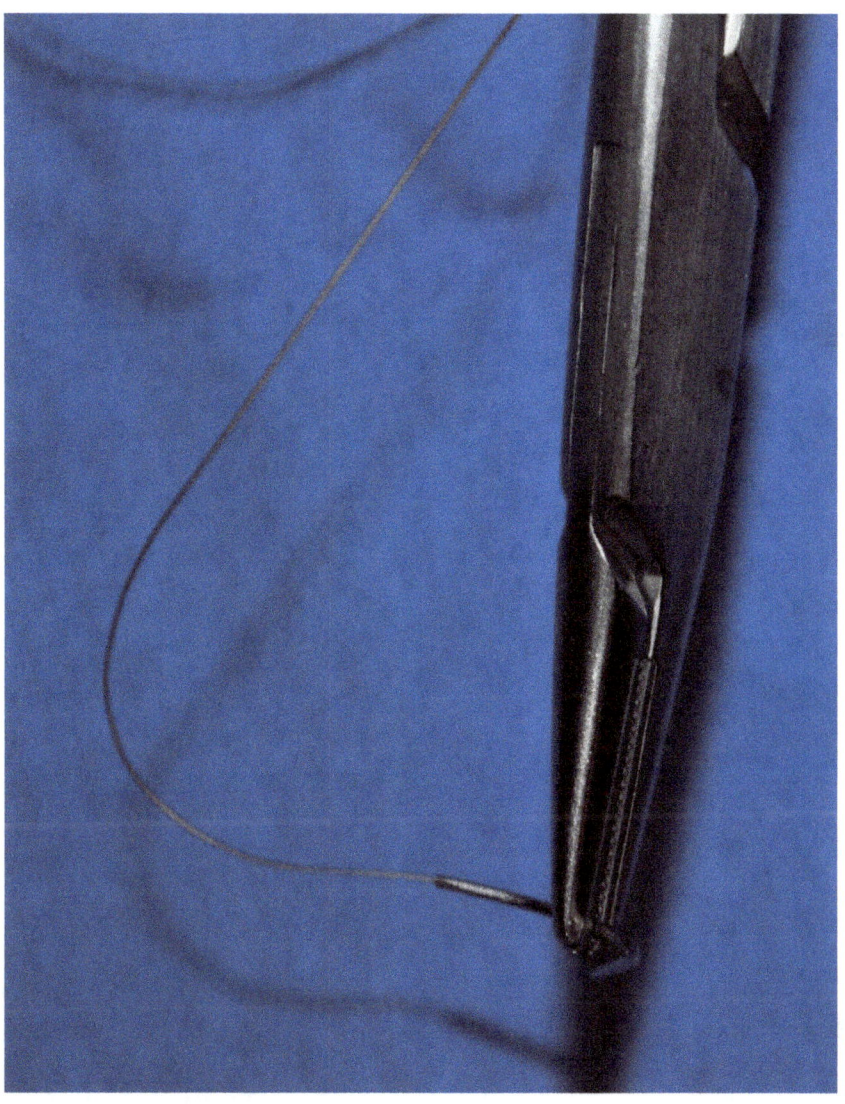

Figure 15.
Correct positioning of the suture needle in the jaws of the needle holder. This is the rear view of a "loaded" needle holder. This is also the view when backhanding the needle to suture away from yourself.

ii. Palm grip

Palming a needle holder is an option for both and right and left hand.

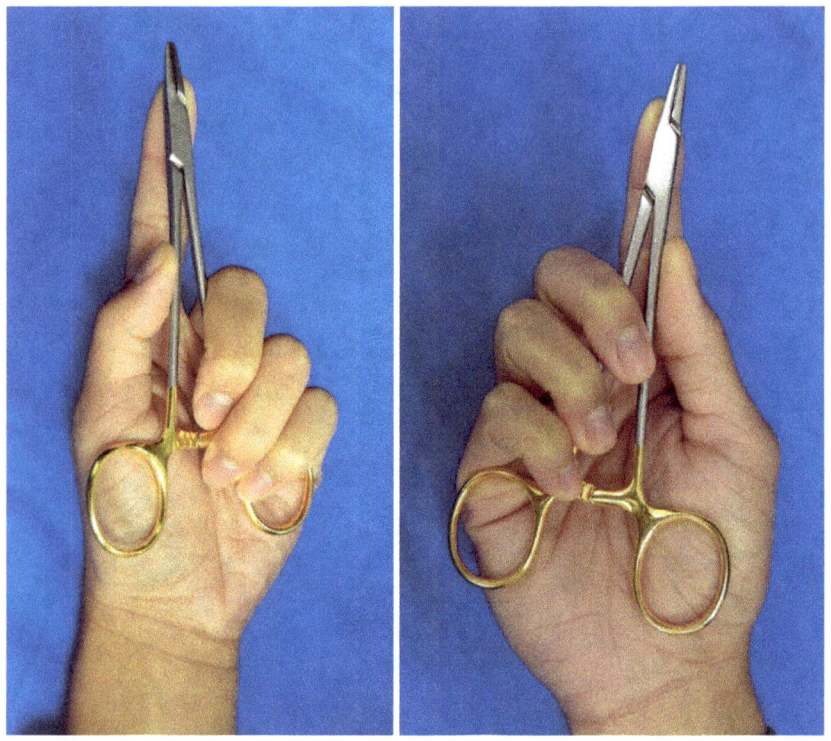

Figure 16.
Palm grip is suitable for left and right hands. This is a useful grip that gives better control of the tip.

iii. 'Palming', as in 'storing' instrument in the palm of the hand

How to palm an instrument: Release the thumb and swivel the instrument around *to* hold in the ulnar side of the palm with your ring finger still through the second ring.

The shank lies along your palm and against your wrist. This way you can have a scissor "at the ready" and swing it around to use. It is possible to use a forceps or another instrument such as a cautery unit, when palming a scissor.

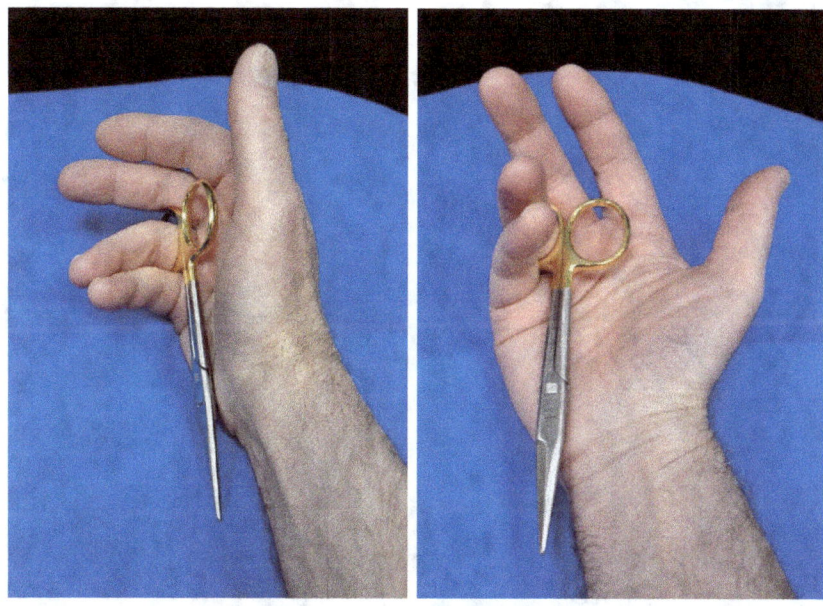

Figure 17.
Palming a scissor. Left: side view. Right: palm view.

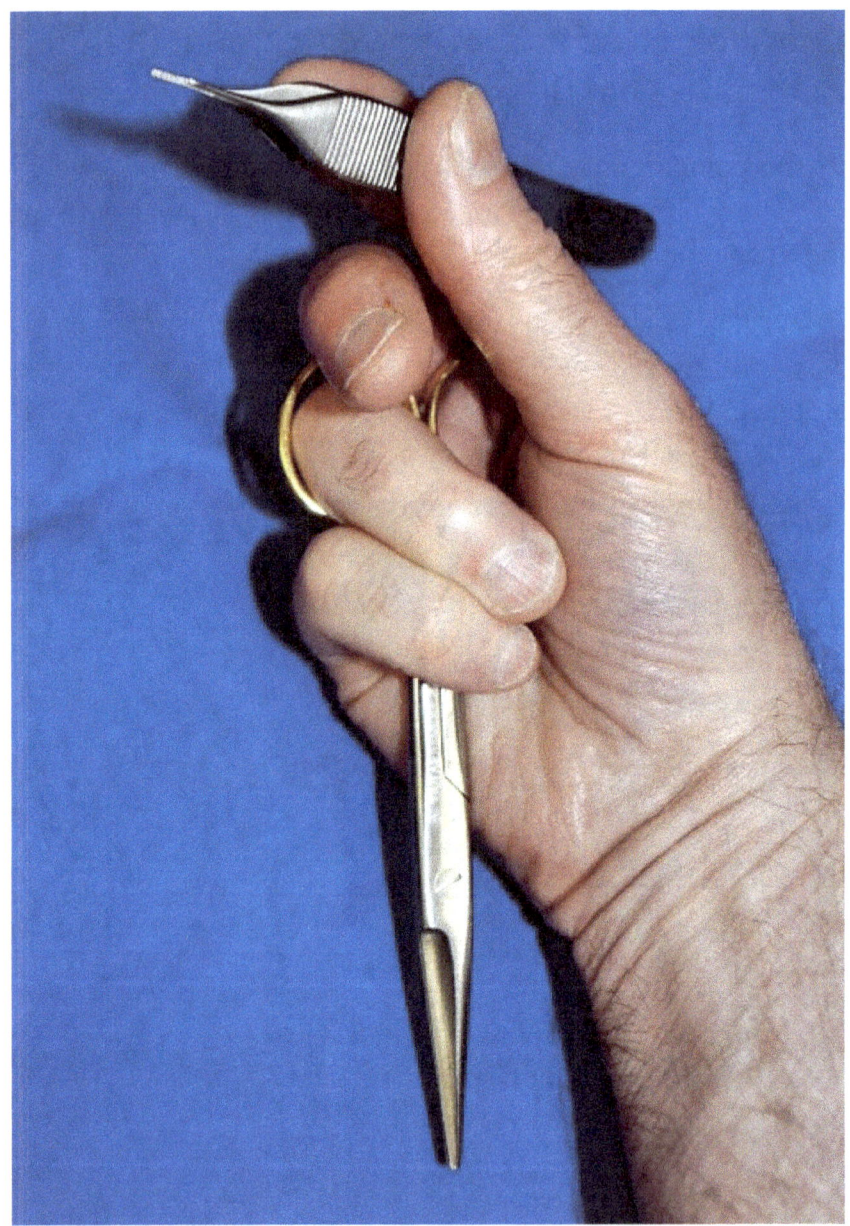

Figure 18.
Using a forceps whilst storing the scissors in your palm.

INSTRUMENTS

B. Holding a spring instrument e.g., forceps.

Toothed Adson forceps are "spring instruments." Compressing the sides of the instrument with the thumb and index finger closes the tips. Releasing the pressure allows the tips to spring open to their resting position. Because pressure is required to keep the tips closed, lengthy use of a forceps may cause cramping in the muscles of the first web space.

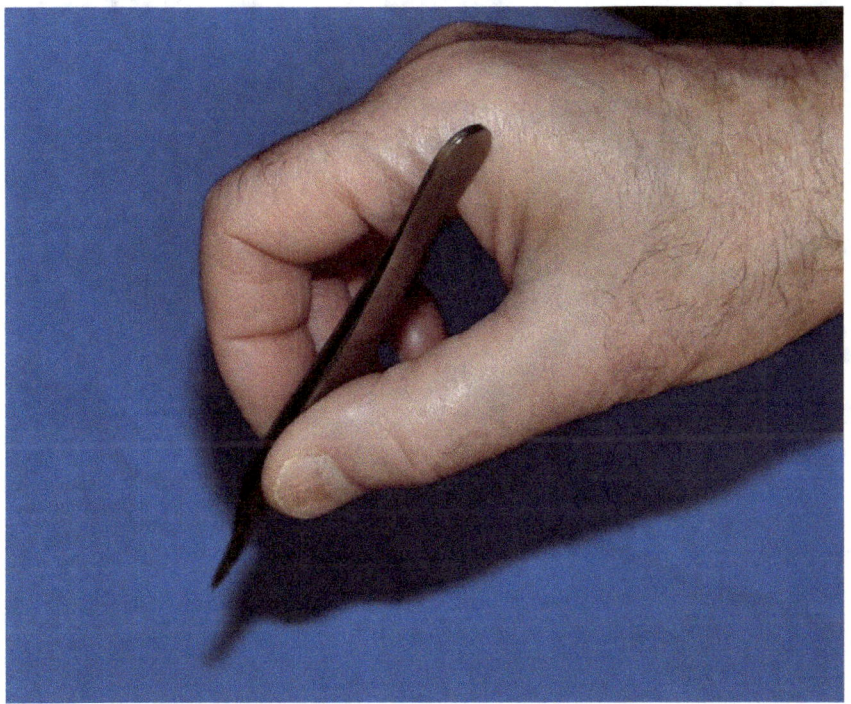

Figure 19.
The base of the forceps rests against the radial side of the first metacarpophalangeal joint in the first web space. The thumb and index finger hold the instrument at the widest part of the handle. Forceps can also be held like a mallet (see below) with the base of the handle hidden in the palm. A spring needle holder may also be held like a forceps in the first web space or within the palm like a mallet.

C. Holding a handled instrument e.g., mallet.

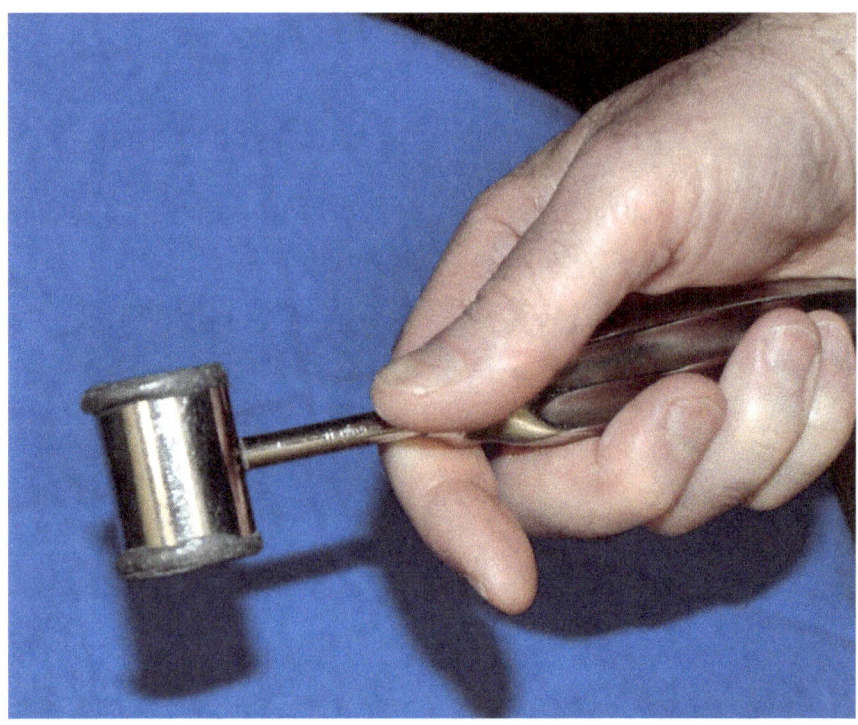

Figure 20.
How to hold a mallet: The handle is nestled inside the palm and is gripped with the middle, ring, and little fingers. The index finger rests under the base of the stem but may also be used to grip the handle. The thumb rests on the top of the stem with head of the mallet ninety degrees to the axis of the thumb.

PLACING SUTURES & KNOT TYING

05

A. Placing sutures

From the needle packet, load a suture needle close to the tip of the needle holder jaws, one half to two thirds along the needle length (two thirds in front and one third behind the jaws). See figures 13 and 14.

You can load a needle single-handed, grasping the needle loosely with the needle holder and then rolling the needle on the jaws until it is correctly positioned, ninety degrees to the jaws.

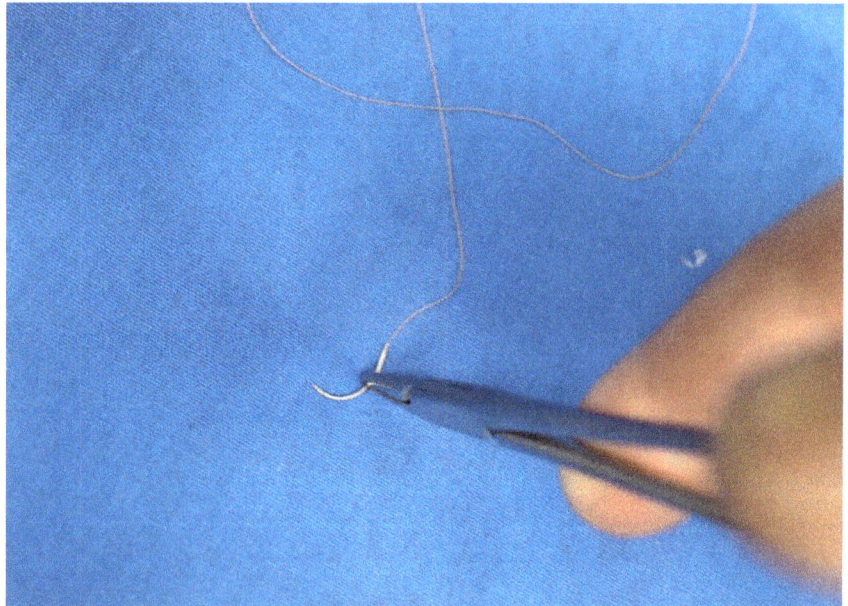

Figure 21.
Alternatively, you can place the jaws at ninety degrees to the surface of the drape and then grasp the needle straight off the drape with the needle holder.

i. Interrupted skin sutures

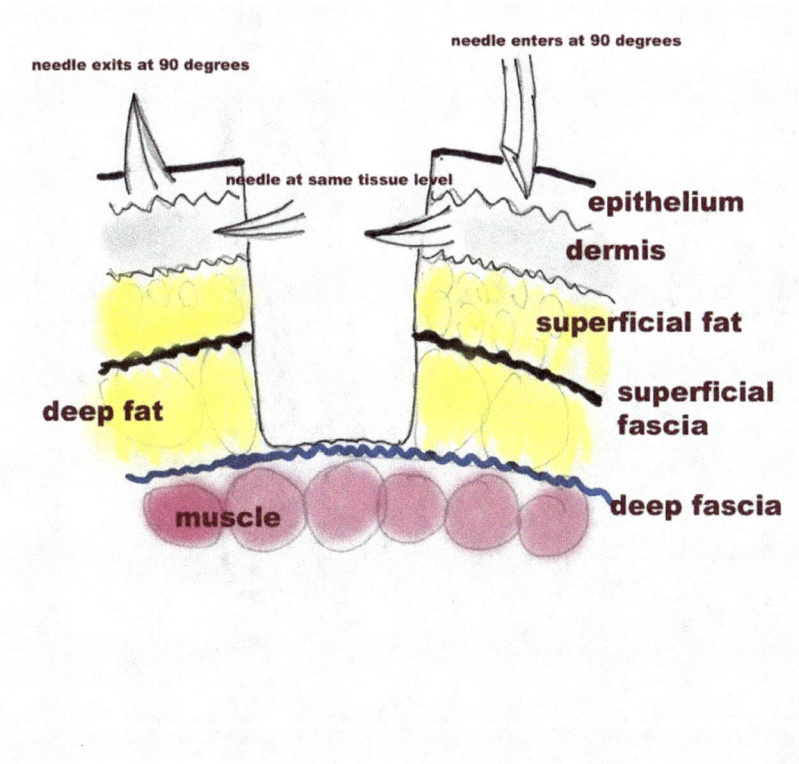

Figure 22.
Incisional tissue layers from superficial to deep (subcuticular stitch passes through the dermis).
1. Epithelium
2. dermis
3. superficial fat with small lobules
4. superficial fascia
5. deep fat with large lobules
6. deep fascia
7. Muscle

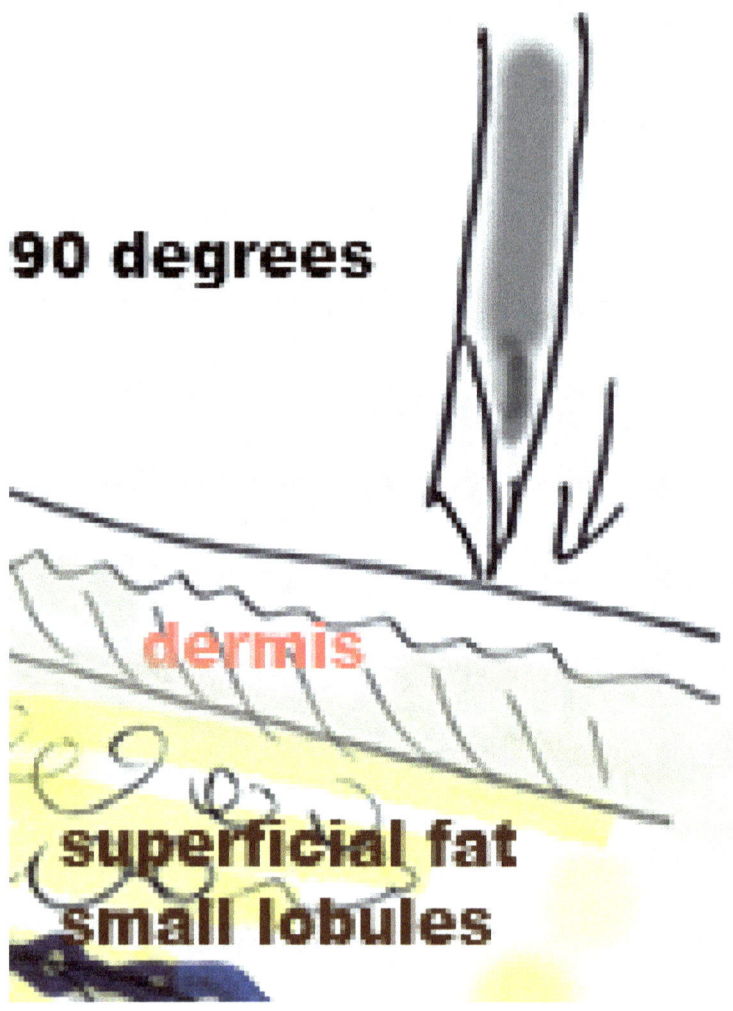

Figure 23.
Pronate your wrist so that the needle point is now 90 degrees to the skin surface, as if you were stabbing the skin.

PLACING SUTURES & KNOT TYING

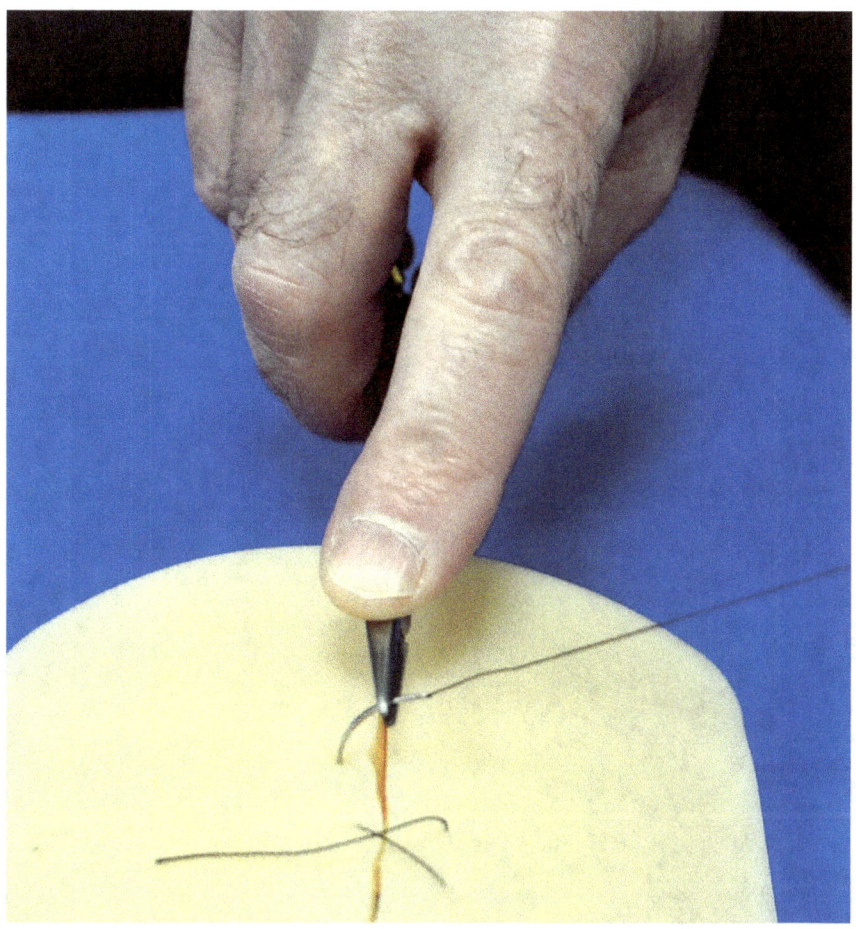

Figure 24.
Pronate the wrist and pierce the first side of the wound 90 degrees to the skin surface. Stab the skin straight through, then partially withdraw the needle and *supinate* the wrist 90 degrees passing through the first side of wound into the open wound.

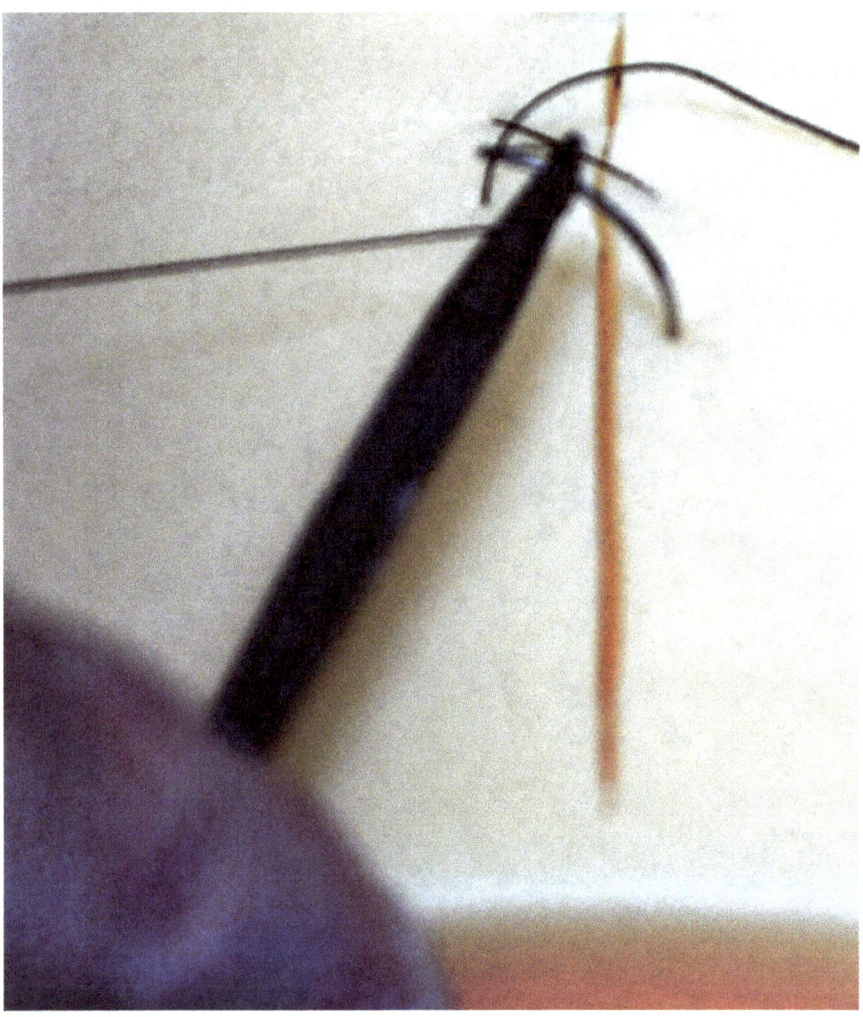

Figure 25.
Piercing the entry side of wound with the needle at 90 degrees to skin. Close-up view.

While still holding the needle in the needle holder, pass the needle through the other side of the wound **at the same depth**. Continue to supinate the wrist until the needle is just beneath the skin surface. Pull the needle back under the skin towards the wound edge, by further supinating the wrist and then exit the skin on the far side, pushing the needle through the skin at 90 degrees to the surface. This technique everts the wound interfaces. Failing to enter and exit at 90 degrees will create an inverted wound edge. (See below).

Using the forceps to apply pressure on the skin surface, over the needle tip, will facilitate the needle's penetration through the surface of the skin on the far side. The same maneuver can be used to deliver and visualize a needle tip when passing the needle within the deep tissue layers as in performing a deep suture.

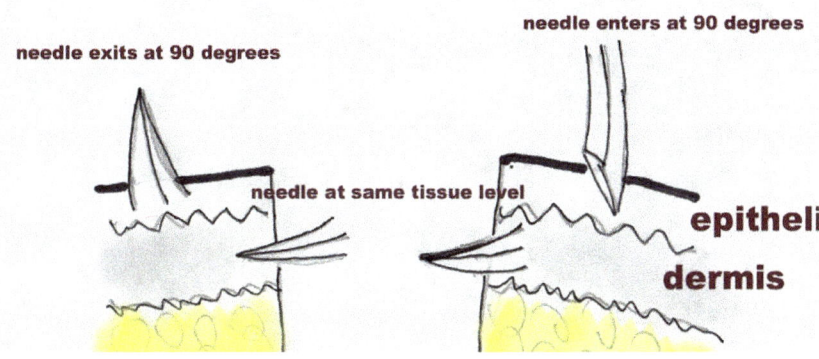

Figure 26.
Diagrammatic view of passing the needle through the wound interface at the same level on both sides of the wound.

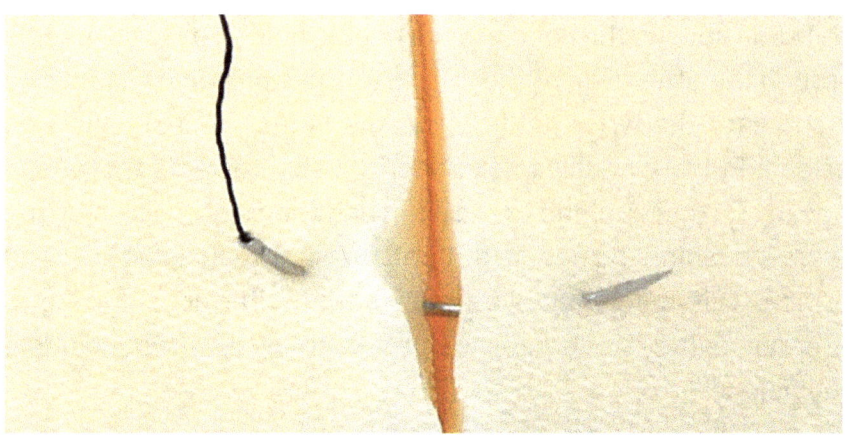

Figure 27.
Passing the needle through the wound interface at the **same level** on both sides of the wound.

PLACING SUTURES & KNOT TYING

If necessary, use two separate bites. After exiting the first side, grasp the needle with the Adson forceps in the open wound whilst still holding the needle in the needle holder. Release the needle holder and reload the needle in the needle holder **before** you release it from the forceps. Now place the second bite from within the open wound *at the same depth* passing through the skin surface on the far side. If you are performing a subcuticular suture, make sure that the needle bites are at the **same tissue level** on each side of the incision.

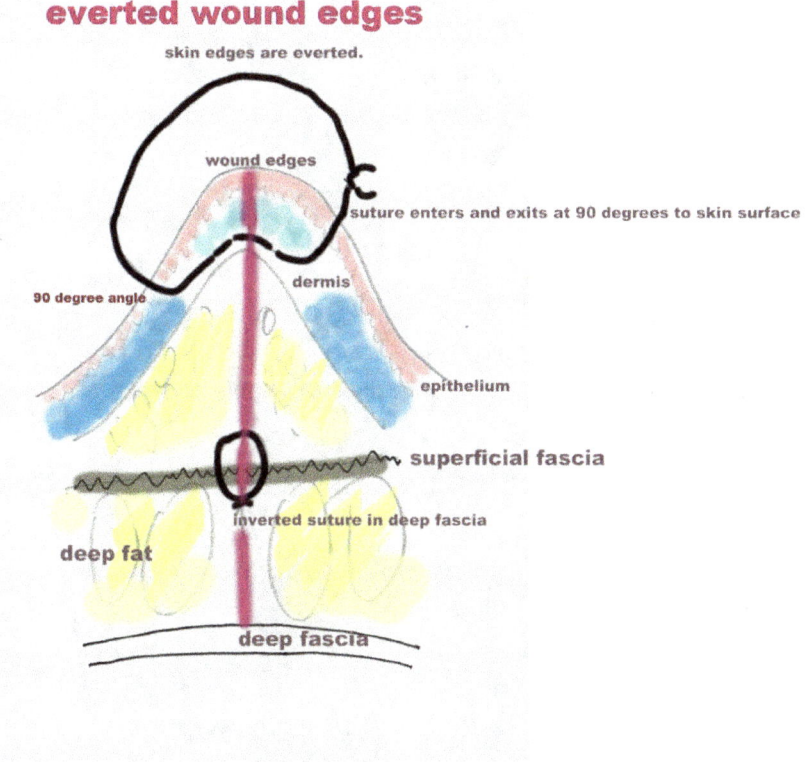

Figure 28.
Eversion of wound edges with entrance and exit of needle body at 90 degrees to skin surface.

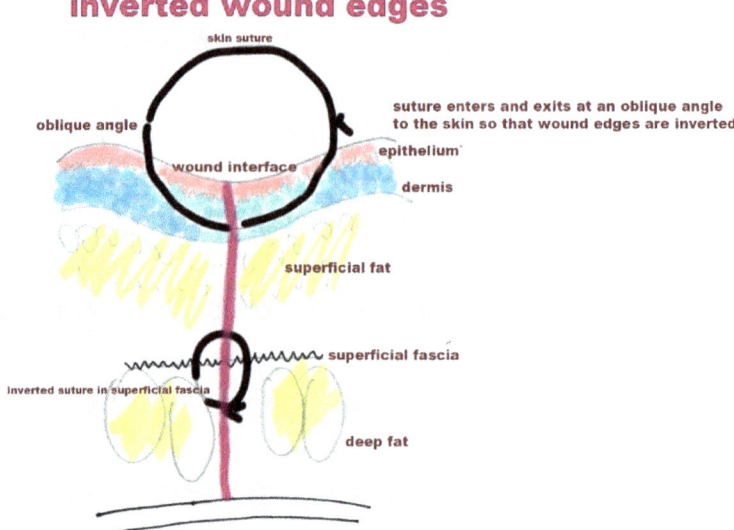

Figure 29.
Inversion of wound edges with entrance and exit of needle body at 45 degrees to skin surface.

PLACING SUTURES & KNOT TYING

ii. Adson toothed forceps tying platform – how to use it

The tying platform is a flat raised area with a gripping surface, which is inserted just above the teeth on each side. A tying platform is essential to be able to grasp the needle as it exits from the tissue. It is exceedingly difficult to grasp the body of the needle without this platform grip

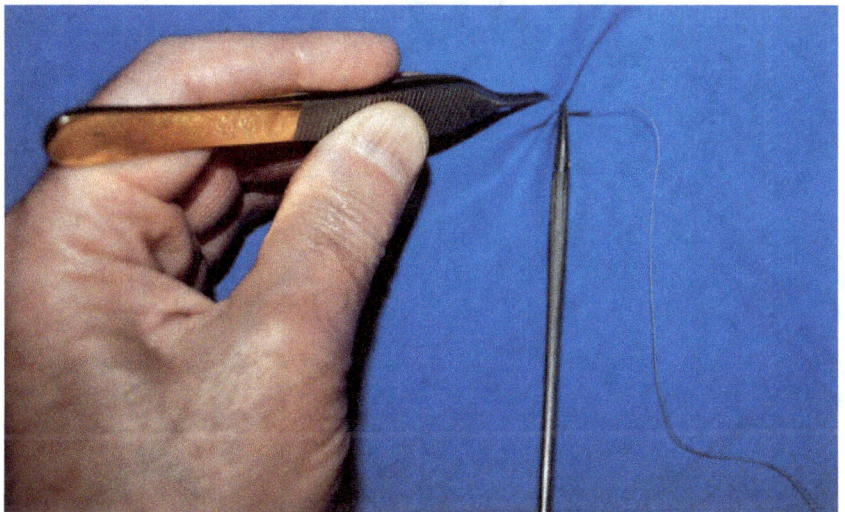

Figure 30.
These are the stages of placing a needle through the incision edge:
1. Grasp the needle as it exits from the wound using the tying platform of the forceps, *whilst still holding the needle in the needle holder on the entrance side of the wound*, as shown above.
2. Release the needle holder on the entrance side.
3. Continue to hold the needle in the forceps.
4. Withdraw the needle from the wound and grasp the needle with the needle holder on the exit side of the wound, at the wound level. (See Figure 31).

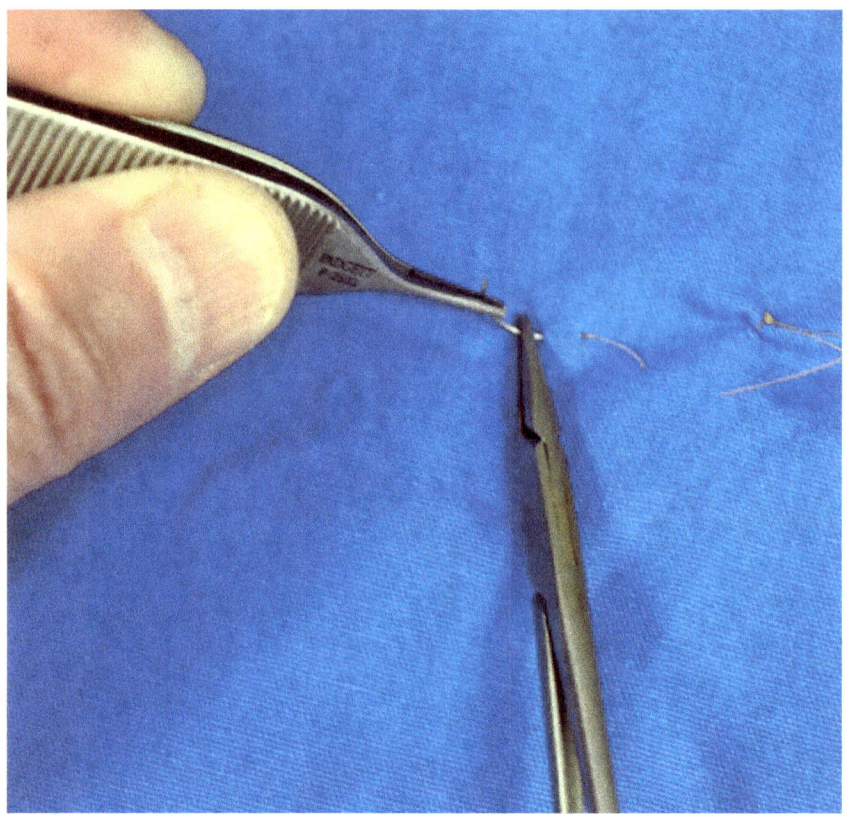

Figure 31.
Grasp the needle with the needle holder before or just as the needle is completely withdrawn. Rest the needle holder on the skin on the **exit** side of the wound.

PLACING SUTURES & KNOT TYING

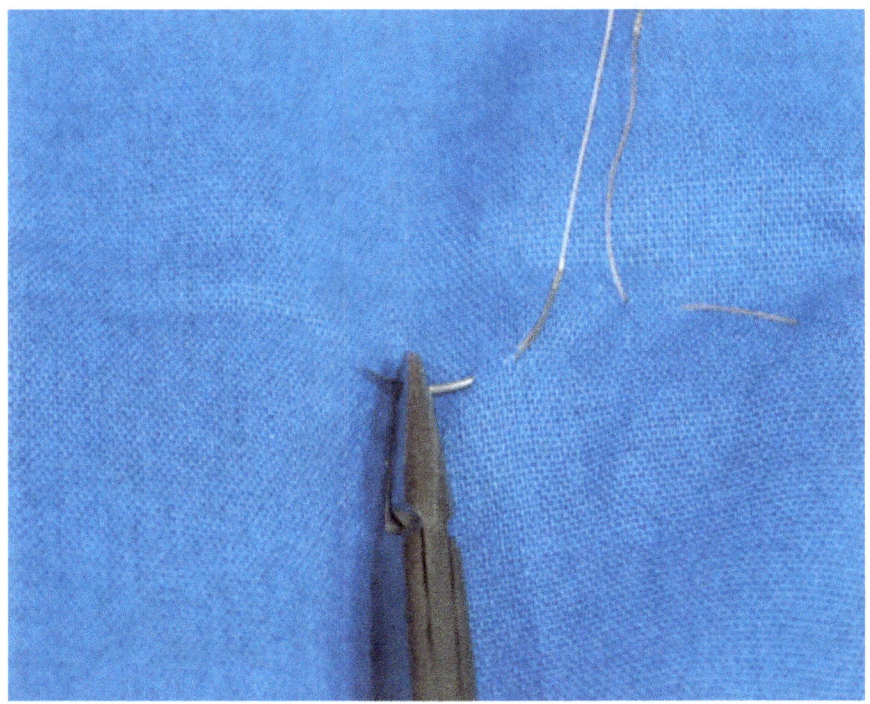

Figure 32.
Release the forceps and pull the needle through with the needle holder. Supinate your wrist as you withdraw the needle to allow the curved needle to exit smoothly.

When performing a subcuticular suture rather than a skin suture, the process is the same, except that you grasp the needle and reload the needle holder each time you take a bite of the subcuticular tissue. Use the same maneuver in deeper tissue sutures such as through Scarpa's fascia, first grasping the needle with the forceps and then reloading the needle in the needle holder before taking the next bite on the opposite side of the wound.

You get faster by eliminating unnecessary maneuvers. Avoid pulling a needle away from the wound before reloading the needle holder. If you do so, before reloading it, then you will have to tighten the suture line with your left hand instead of using the ring and little fingers of the right hand (see Figure 33).

iii. Tightening the suture and closing the wound edges.

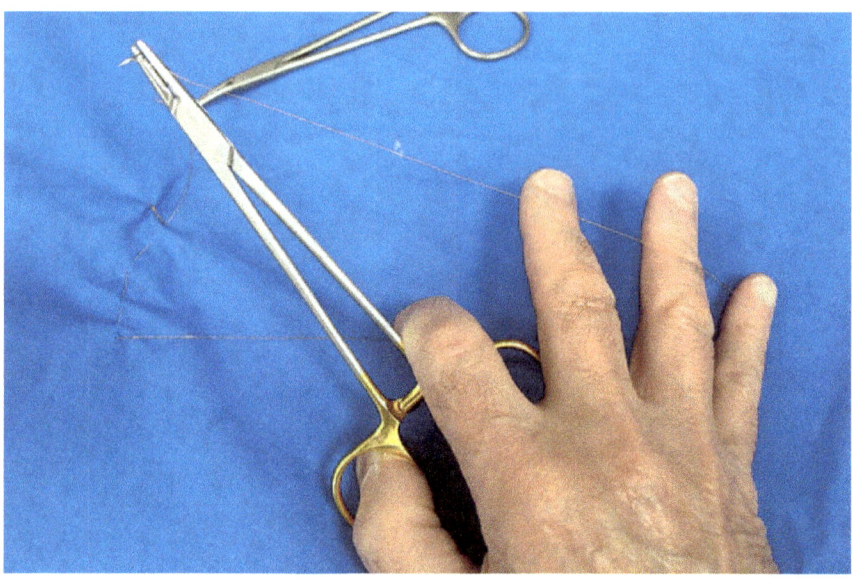

Figure 33.
When performing a subcuticular or a running suture, you can tighten the preceding loop with the ring and little fingers of the right hand. An alternative to this technique is to use the left hand to pull on the suture loop. Do **NOT** use the loaded needle holder to tighten the loop, as this will likely cause the needle and the suture to separate.

The disadvantage of pulling the needle away from the wound is that it forces you to reload the needle by holding the needle in your left hand and reloading it into the needle holder. Furthermore, you have now withdrawn needle and the needle holder out of the surgical field (with its optimal lighting), and your eyes must accommodate to the lower light. All these separate actions will slow you down and may also increase tremor, because your hands are no longer stabilized on the patient (see below).

B. Hand tremor – how to reduce it

Surgeons and assistants may have a shaky hand or a tremor. To reduce this, rest your hands directly on the skin. Rest your hand on the patient to limit your tremor so that only your hand beyond the wrist or the metacarpo-phalangeal (MP) joints is unsupported.

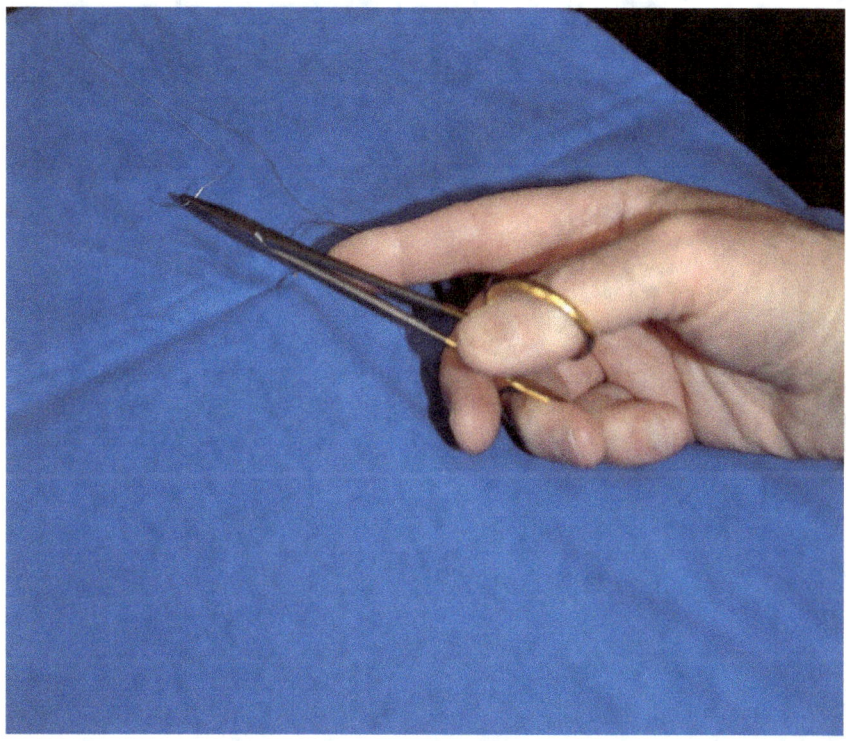

Figure 34.
Hand resting on patient is stable from MP joints.

KIRWAN'S OPERATION ROOM TECHNIQUES

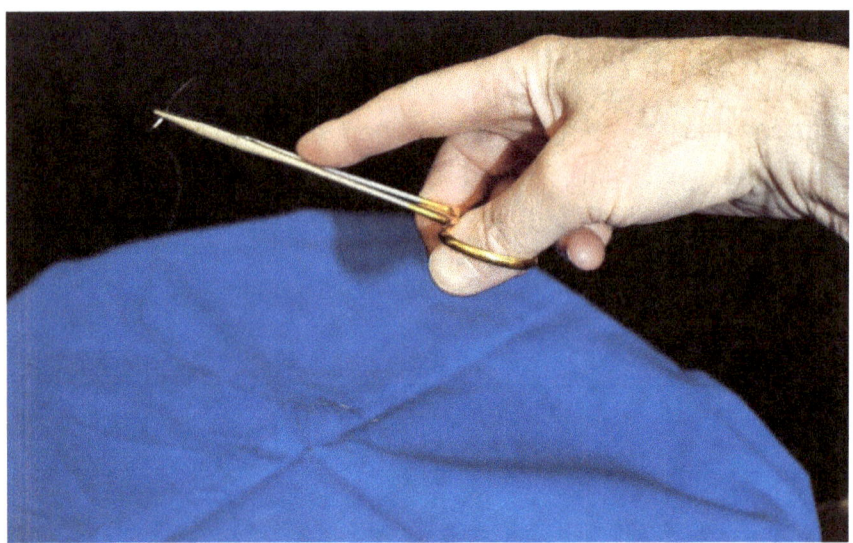

Figure 35.
Hand not resting. Nearest point of stability is shoulder. This is the least stable position.

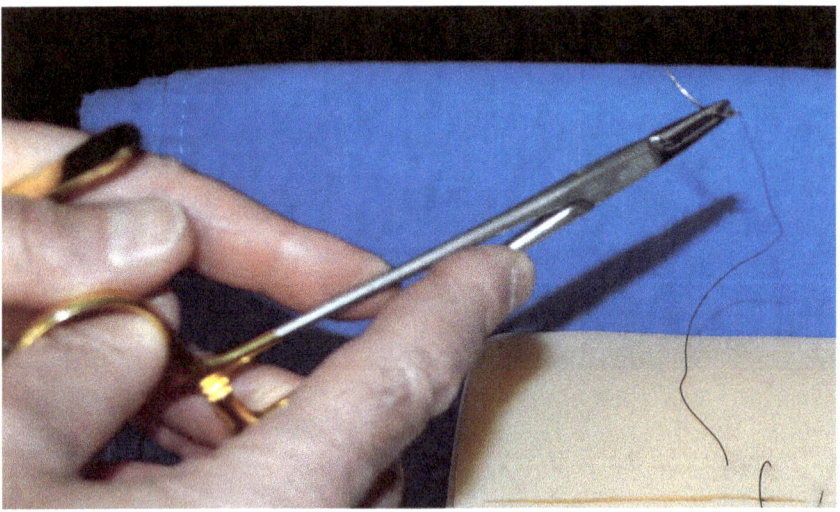

Figure 36.
You can stabilize your right hand with your left hand.
You can also rest your elbows if you cannot rest your wrists. As an alternative, tuck your elbows into your sides.

C. Knot tying

General comments

Each clockwise or counterclockwise loop of a suture is called a "throw." The term "knot" may sometimes be used interchangeably with the term "throw." The final combination of throws is a "knot."

There are many ways to tie a knot, just as there are many ways to tie shoelaces or a tie. In this section, I'll explain the way I do it. If it works for you, then use it. Whichever technique you learn, the most important aim is to achieve a facility at performing one-handed and two-handed knots, so that it is as easy as tying your shoes laces. You should not have to think about it. When you have reached that point, you have successfully learned the technique. On the other hand, you should always be aware of how you tie a knot because from time to time you will have to focus on the mechanics of tying, to make sure that the knot is secure.

In the illustrations below for hand tying, there are certain conventions. The red suture is the **short end,** and the white suture is the **long end**. For instrument ties, the red tsuture is always shorter. The white suture usually has the needle attached. Sometimes, the needle is a "pull-off" type, meaning the needle is pulled off the suture with the needle holder prior to tying the knot. Sometimes the needle is simply removed by cutting the suture before tying the knot. When performing hand ties without the needle attached, both ends may be cut to the same length. For example, when securing a drain or when ligating a blood vessel. The right or left index finger may be used to guide the knot down whilst holding the other end taught.

Suture types

Different sutures have different knot tying characteristics. Braided sutures form more secure knots. Synthetic monofilament suture such as Nylon or Prolene are more likely to unravel and therefore requires a minimum of four to five throws. Use half-hitches unless you specifically require square knots. With a square knot, a **minimum** of three throws is required to make a knot secure. The first throw is often a surgeon's knot. For half-hitches, use four to five throws or more depending on how secure you want the knot to be.

When performing instrument ties, the short end remains in one place, 180 degrees opposite. See Figure 45. Do not cross your hands unless you want a square knot.

One advantage of a half-hitch, either as a hand or instrument tie, is that the first and second throws can be tightened down together using the index finger, before applying additional throws. In contrast, an initial square throw will be immobile and cannot be slipped down or made tighter when tightening the second throw.

Knots for interrupted sutures should all be placed on the same side of incision and the sutures should be inserted at even intervals. There are exceptions, but this is a good rule. It looks neater and more professional. Do not strangulate knots down. It will cause tissue necrosis. Tissue swelling after wound closure will always increase suture tightness.

When creating a square knot rather than a half-hitch, you will need to cross your hands after the first or second throw, depending on the direction of the knot. (See below) A surgeon's knot is usually two clockwise loops which are laid flat and square.

PLACING SUTURES & KNOT TYING

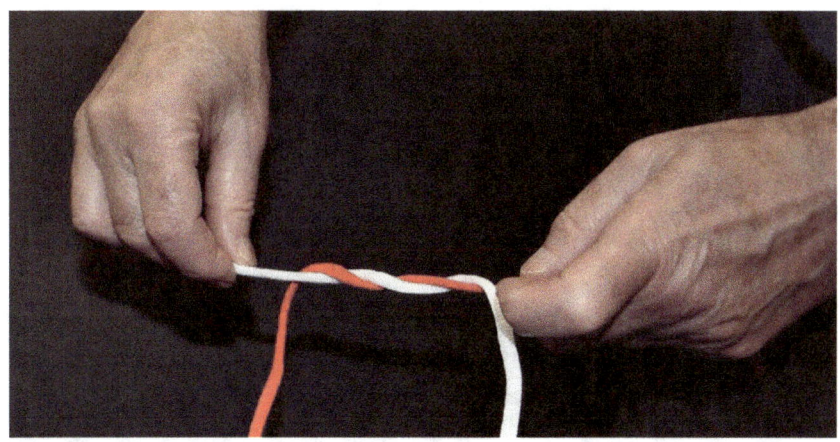

See Figure 37.
Surgeon's knot.

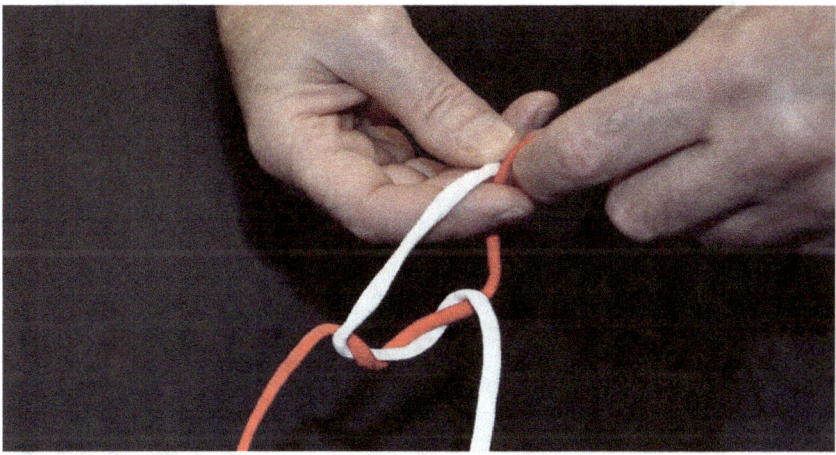

Figure 38.
A single square throw in the opposite direction will lock the knot. Surgeon's knots (two-handed ties and instrument ties) are important when you are closing tissues under tension or securing a drain and want to prevent a knot from slipping. See also Figure 46.

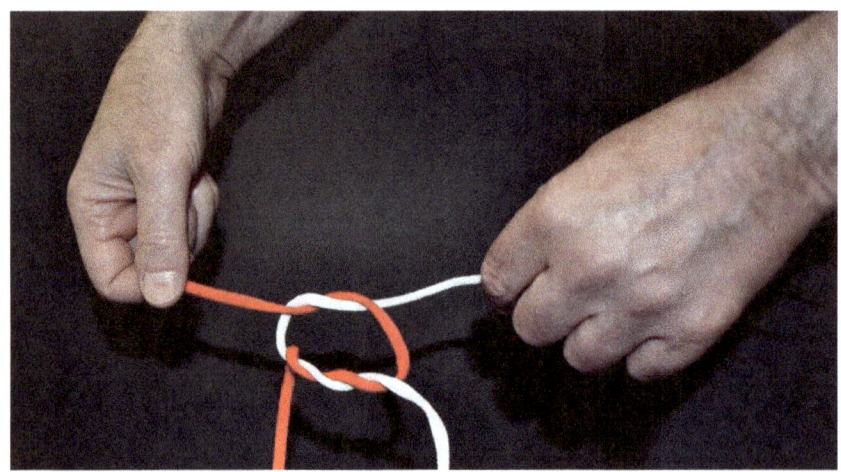

Figure 39.
A single square throw in the opposite direction locks the knot. See Figure 46 also for the instrument tie version.

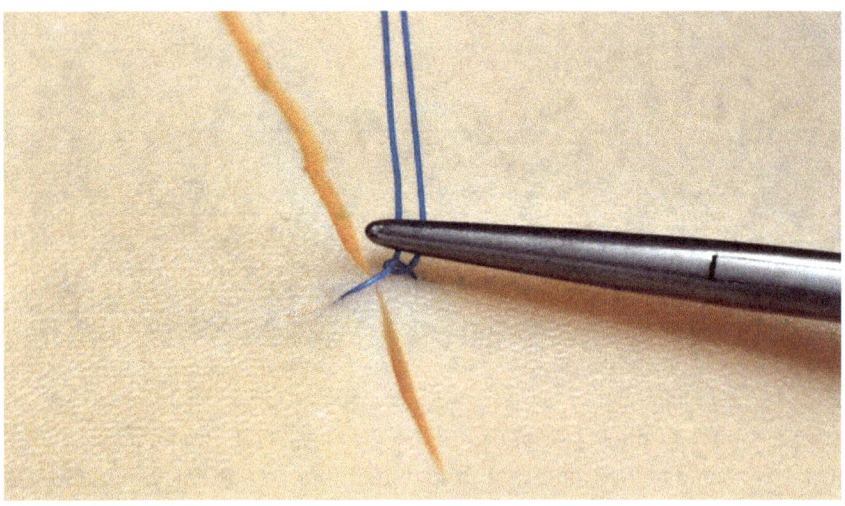

Figure 40.
An alternative to a surgeon's knot is to have the assistant clamp both ends of the suture with a needle holder after the first throw and before making the second throw. The assistant then releases the jaws of the needle holder as the second throw comes down to lock the first.

i. Instrument tie

Instrument ties are the preferred method of suture tying, they are generally faster and more economical of suture material.

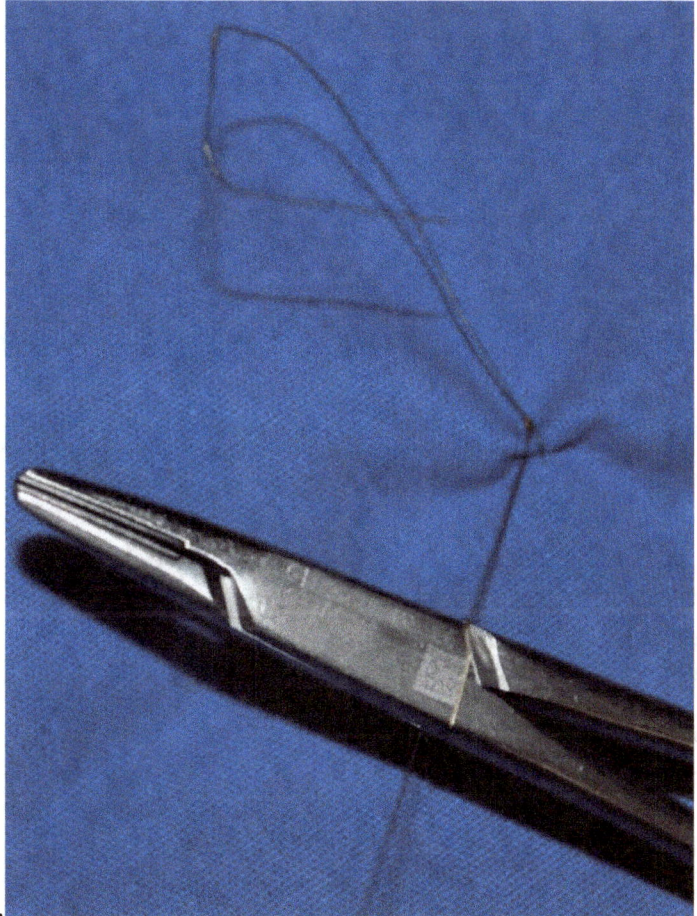

Figure 41.
Instrument tie. Wrap the suture clockwise around the hinge of the needle holder and then grasp the short end in the jaws of the needle holder. Pull the short end through the loop you have created. If the suture is a deep suture with an inverted or upside-down knot, the first throw is counterclockwise and the second clockwise, and so on.

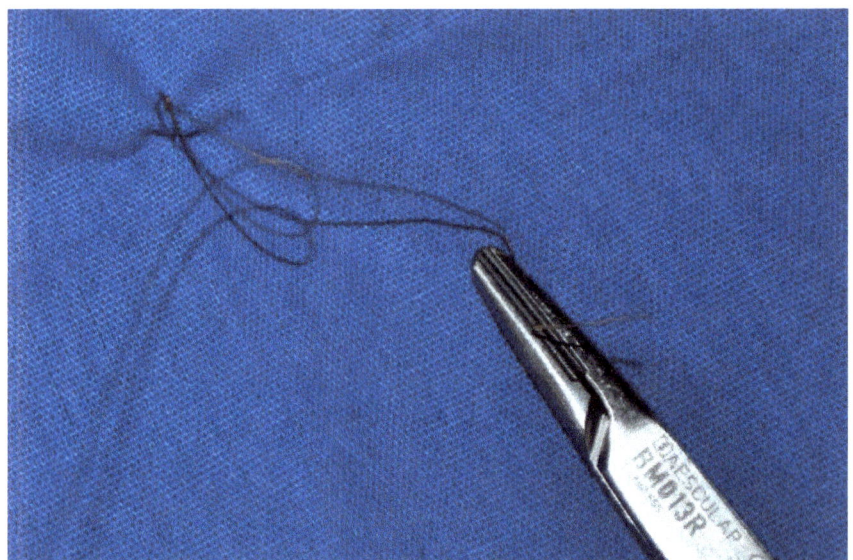

Figure 42.
Pull the short end through the loop and return the short end to the opposite side of incision (Figure 43). Repeat the same maneuver in a counter-clockwise direction. Perform four to five throws, alternating between clockwise and counterclockwise loops.

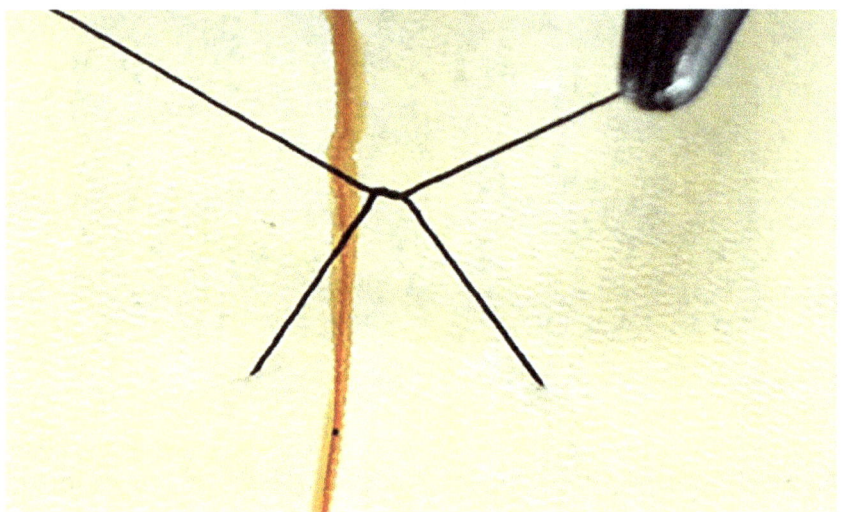

Figure 43.
Square knot, first single throw of an instrument tie.

PLACING SUTURES & KNOT TYING

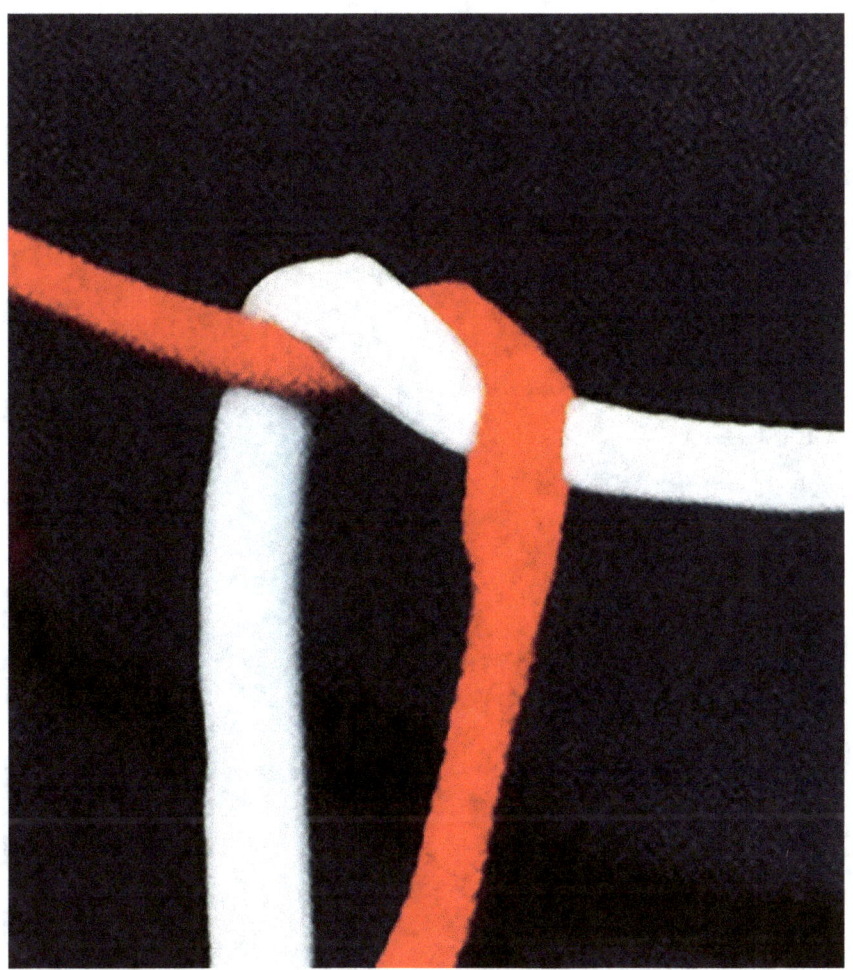

Figure 44.
Square knot, close up view.

KIRWAN'S OPERATION ROOM TECHNIQUES

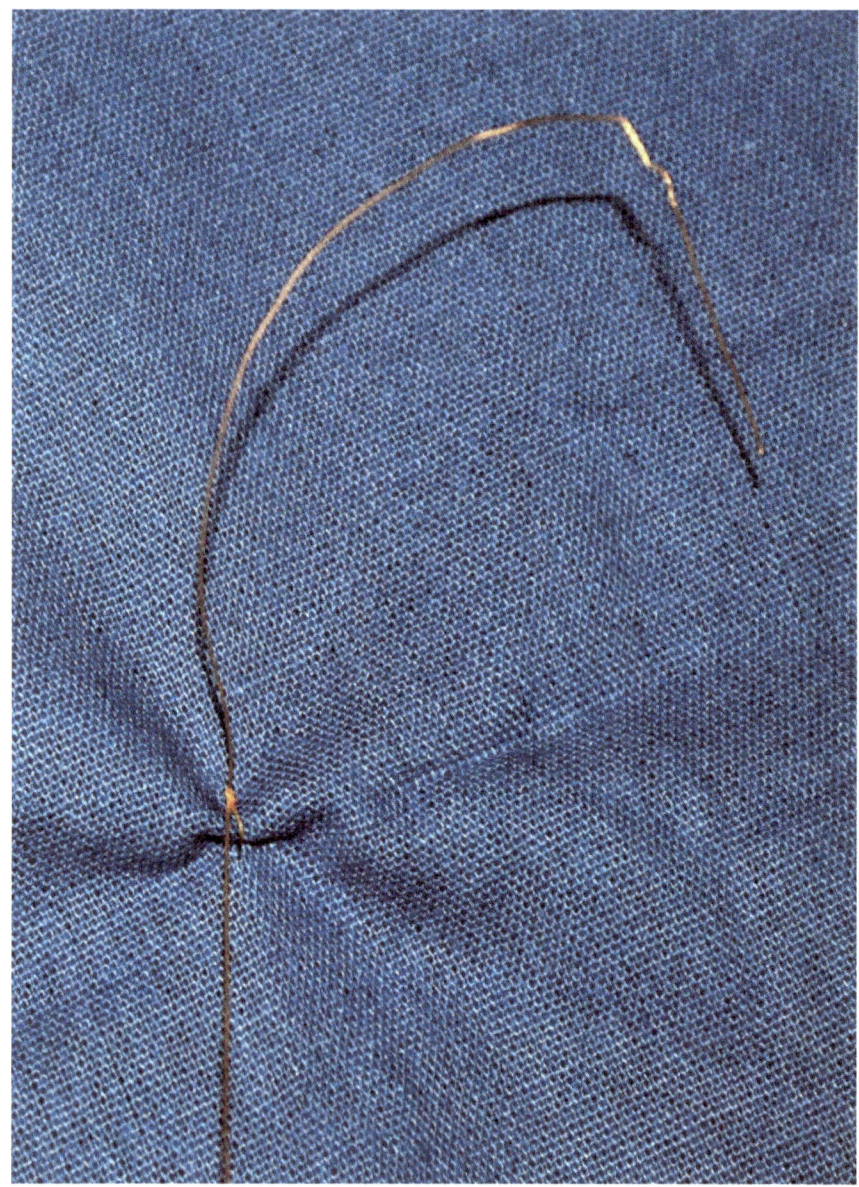

Figure 45.
The first throw is pulled snugly, and the short end is placed on the opposite side of the wound. The second loop is counterclockwise, again returning the short end of the suture to the far side. Do **not** cross your hands unless you wish to create a square knot.

PLACING SUTURES & KNOT TYING

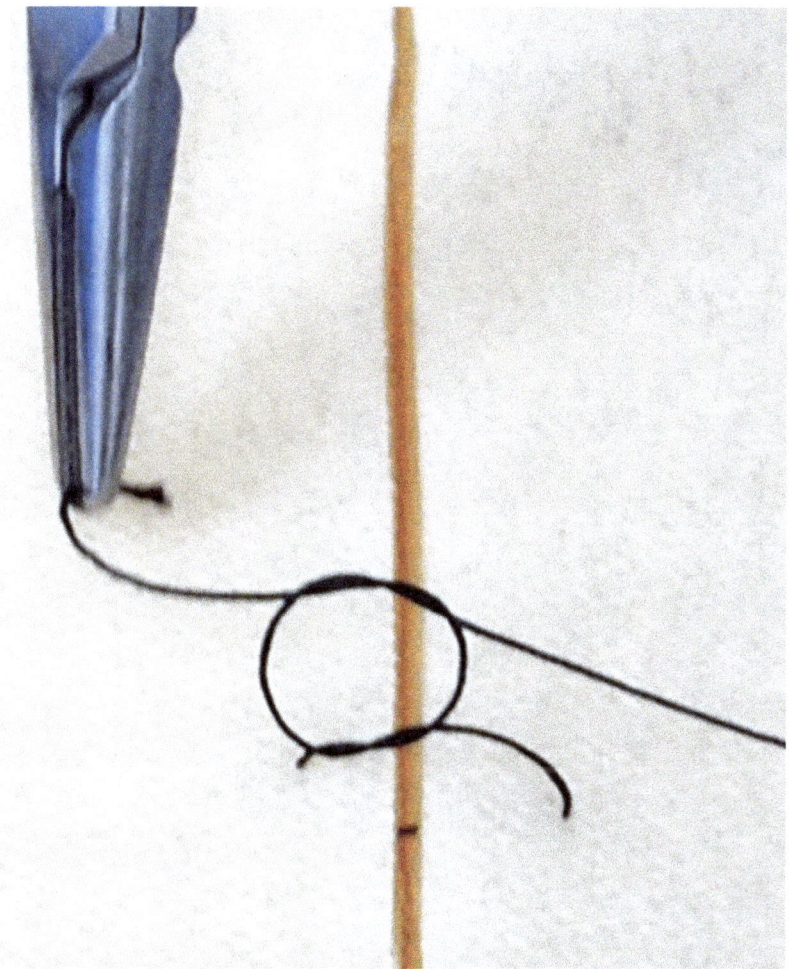

Figure 46.
A surgeon's knot is created with two clockwise loops around the needle holder. After this is pulled down, a counterclockwise loop is made to create a single square locking throw which is tightened down on the surgeon's knot. The hands are crossed to keep the knot square.

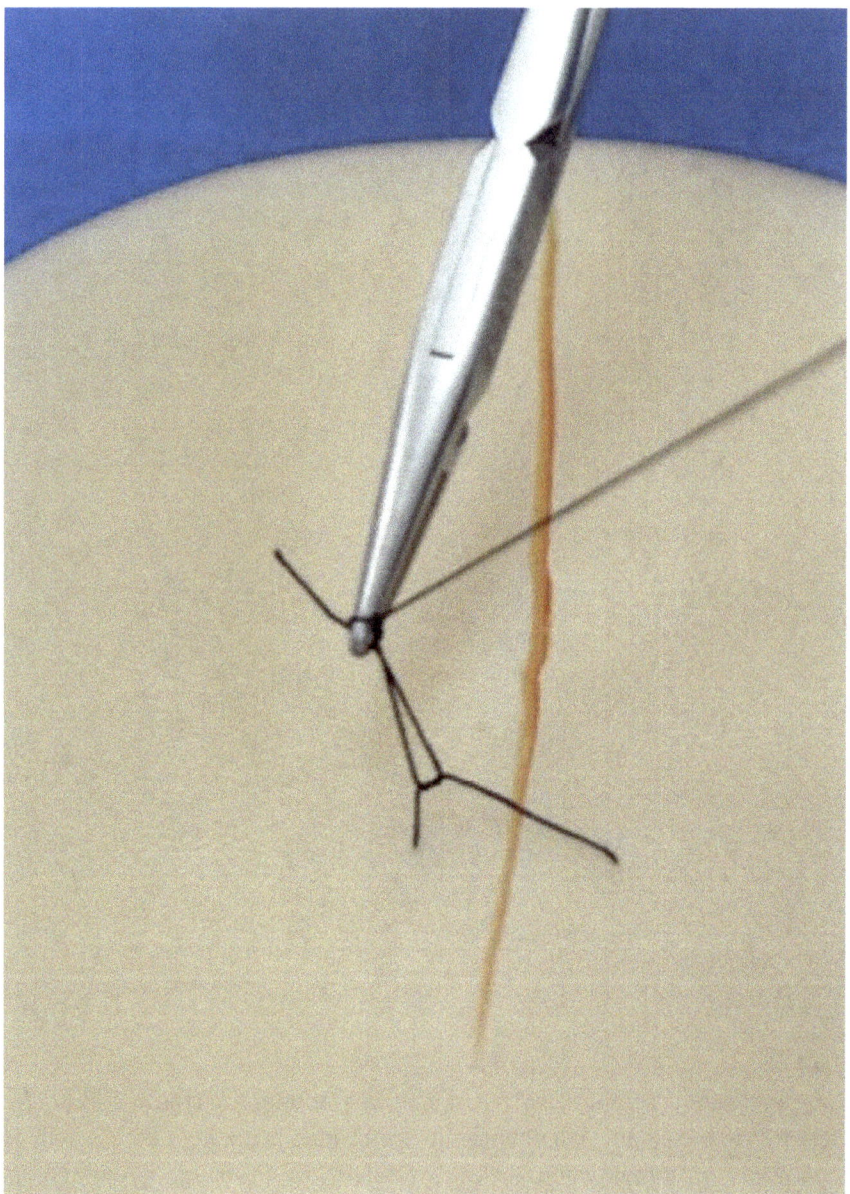

Figure 47.
When the hands are not crossed the knot is a half hitch. A "*post*" is the long end of the suture which is pulled to the right in this picture. The long end, or post, is looped around the needle holder and the short end is then grasped with the needle holder. The hands are not crossed.

PLACING SUTURES & KNOT TYING

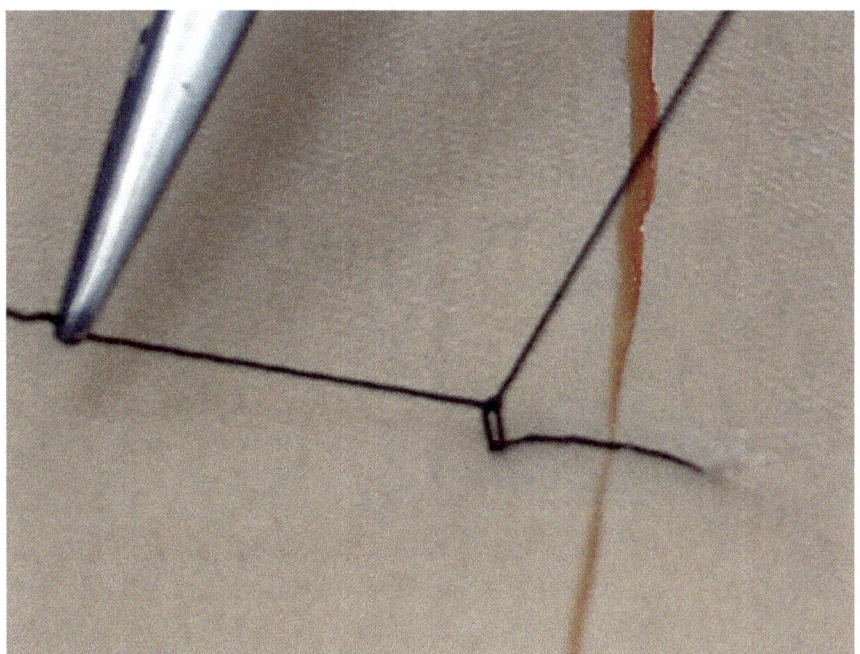

Figure 48.
Two half-hitches on same post can be slipped down and locked. The post is shown here on right. The post can be alternated to create a reversed half-hitch, which is less likely to slip. However multiple half-hitches will also create a secure non-slip knot.

ii. Hand tie

a. One-handed knot

These are the steps to tying a one-handed knot.

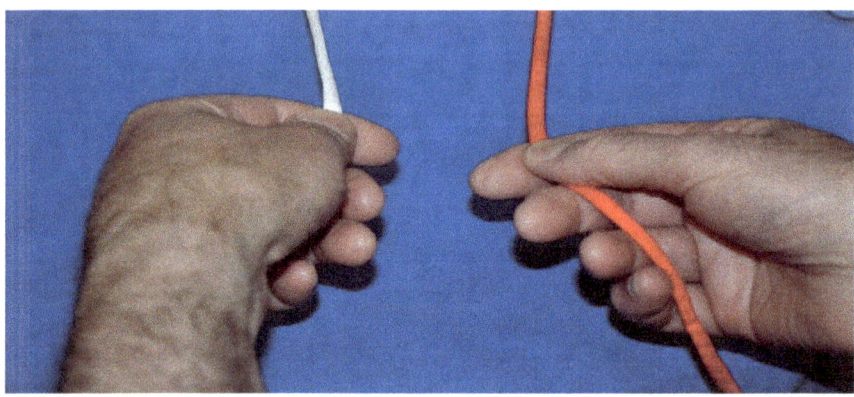

Figure 49.
Step 1. Hold the ends of the suture towards you, using the thumb and index finger of each hand. Hold the short red end with the right hand and the long white end with your left hand. The long end is usually the end with the needle attached.

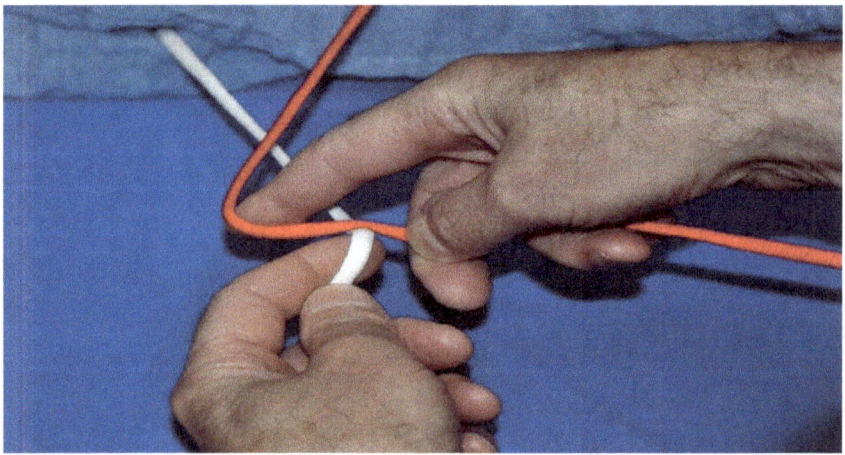

Figure 50.
Step 2. Using the index finger of your right hand, pronate your wrist and cross the short red end in front of the long white end whilst pinching the short red end between the right thumb and middle finger.

PLACING SUTURES & KNOT TYING

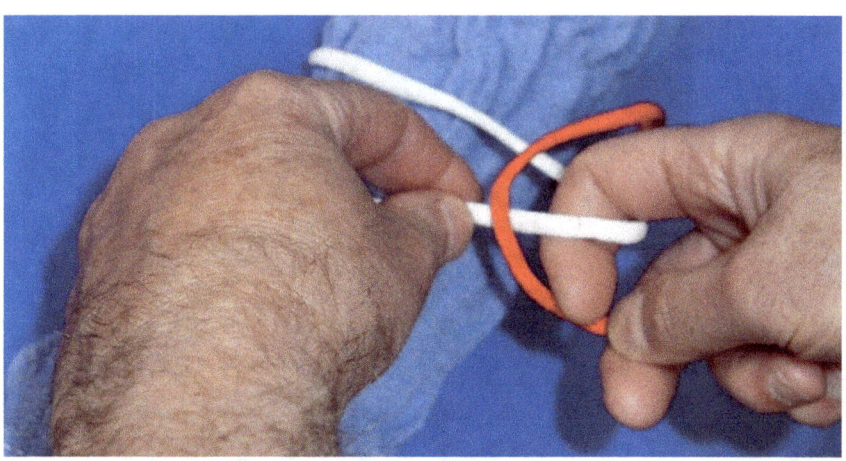

Figure 51.

Step 3. Allow the white end to relax so you can flex and pronate your right wrist, then curl the right index in front of and around the long white end and over and on top of the short red end, which is held between the thumb and middle finger of the right hand.

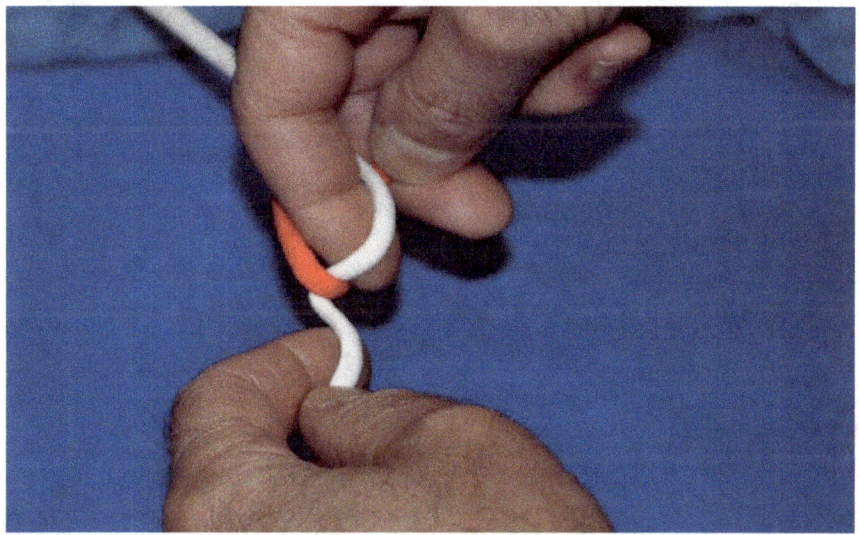

Figure 52.

Step 4. Now extend the tip of the right index, bringing the short red end forwards with the red end on the back of the right index whilst still holding the short red end between the thumb and middle finger of the right hand.

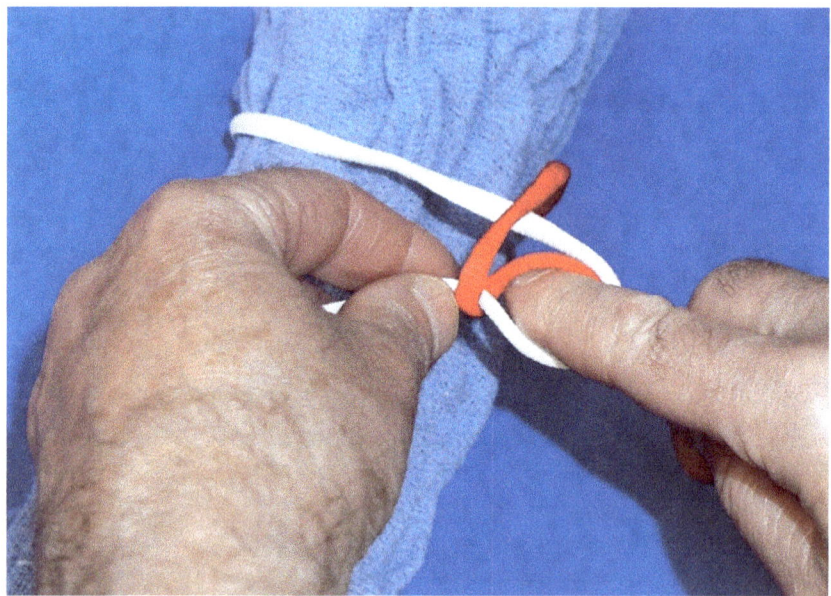

Figure 53.

Step 5. Continue bringing the red end forward with the back of the extended right index finger, whilst still holding the red suture between the thumb and middle finger of the right hand.

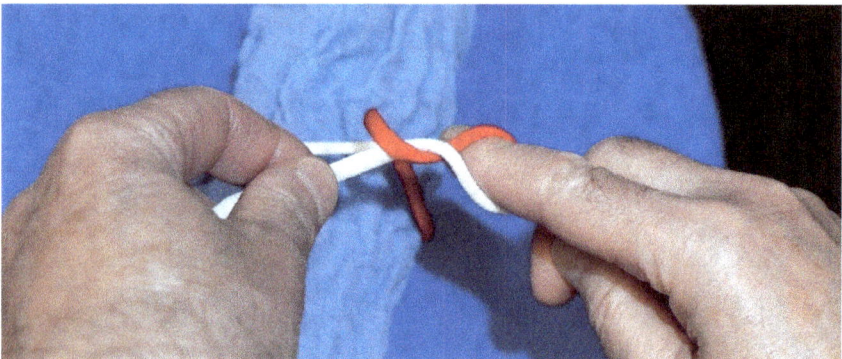

Figure 54.

Step 6. Now, dorsiflex (extend) the right wrist with the straight index finger. These two maneuvers pull the short red end forward as shown, allowing it to wrap around the long end in a counterclockwise direction.

PLACING SUTURES & KNOT TYING

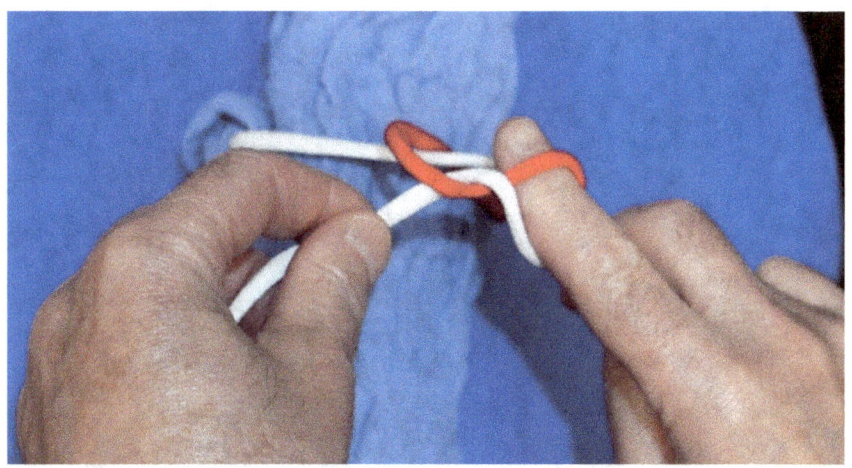

Figure 55.
Step 7. Continue to dorsiflex (extend) the right wrist.

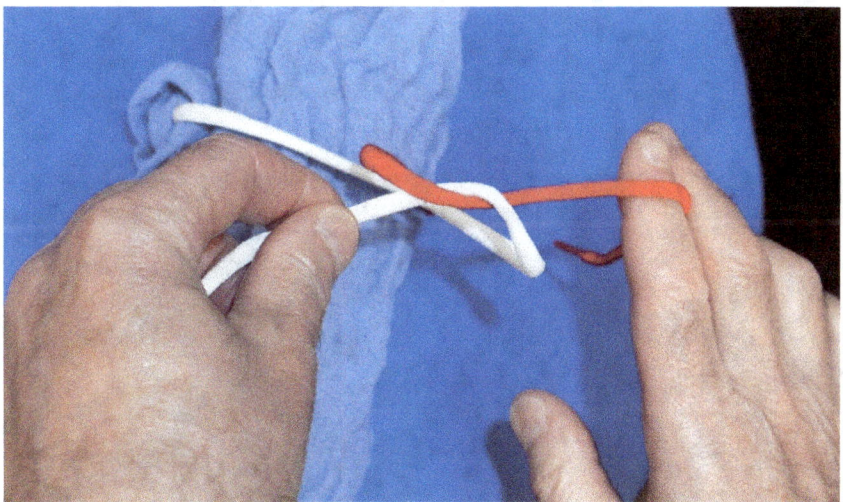

Figure 56.
Step 8. Pull the short red end through the knot by moving your right wrist further to the right releasing the red end from between the thumb and middle finger.

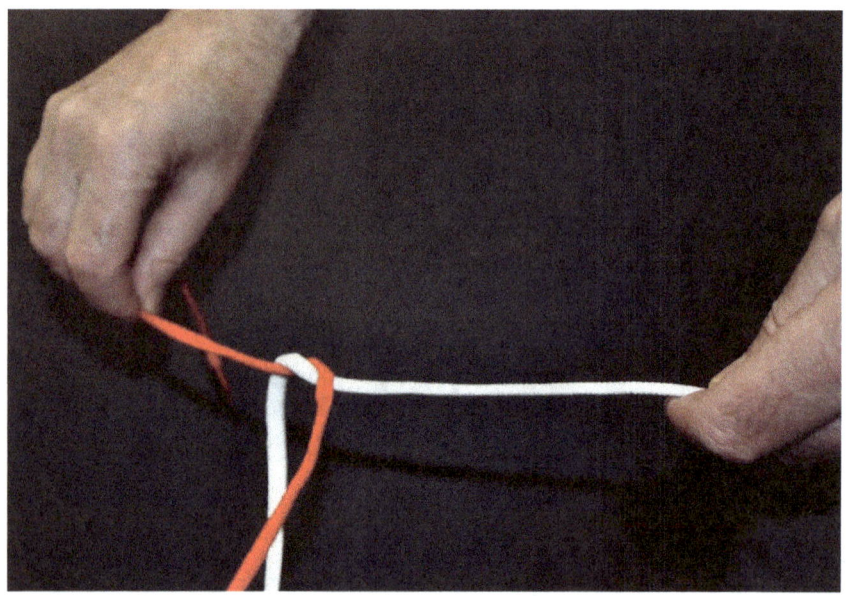

Figure 57.
Step 9. As you pull the short end through, on the back of the index finger, grasp it between your right thumb and index finger as shown.

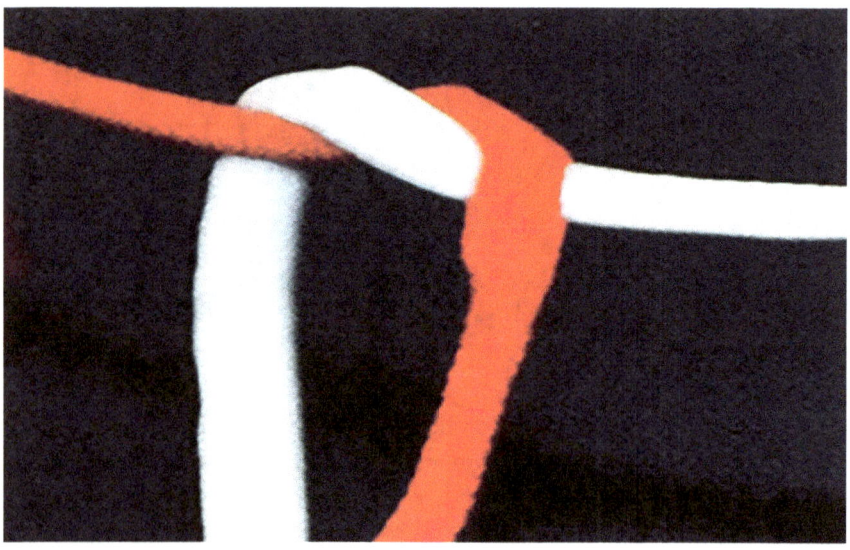

Figure 58.
Step 9. Pulling the short end through, creating a single square knot.

PLACING SUTURES & KNOT TYING

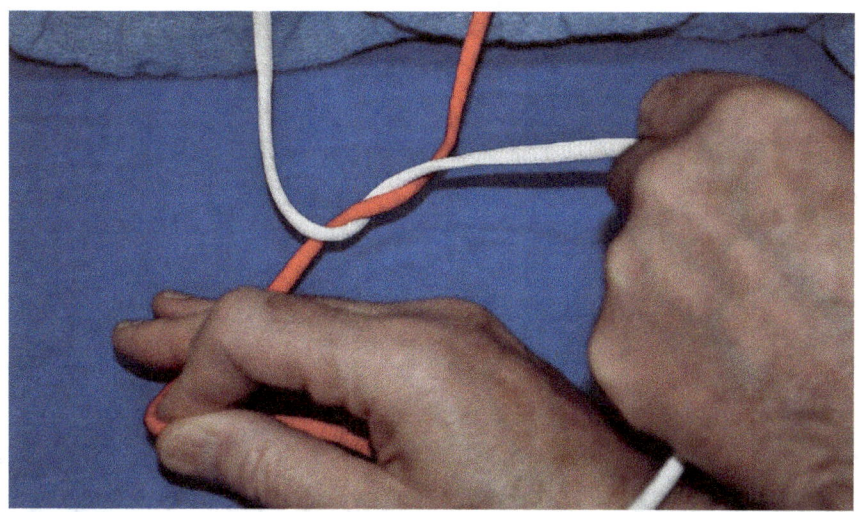

Figure 59.

Step 10. Cross your left hand in front of the right whilst still holding the suture ends. The knot will now lay flat and square.

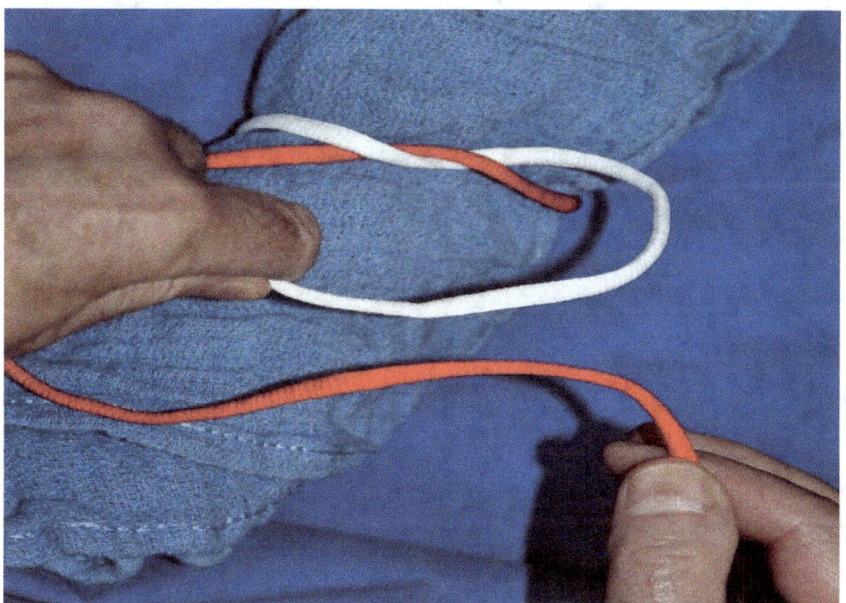

Figure 60.

Step 11. The second throw is in the opposite (clockwise) direction. Keep hold of the short red end in the right hand and bring the right hand back to your right.

KIRWAN'S OPERATION ROOM TECHNIQUES

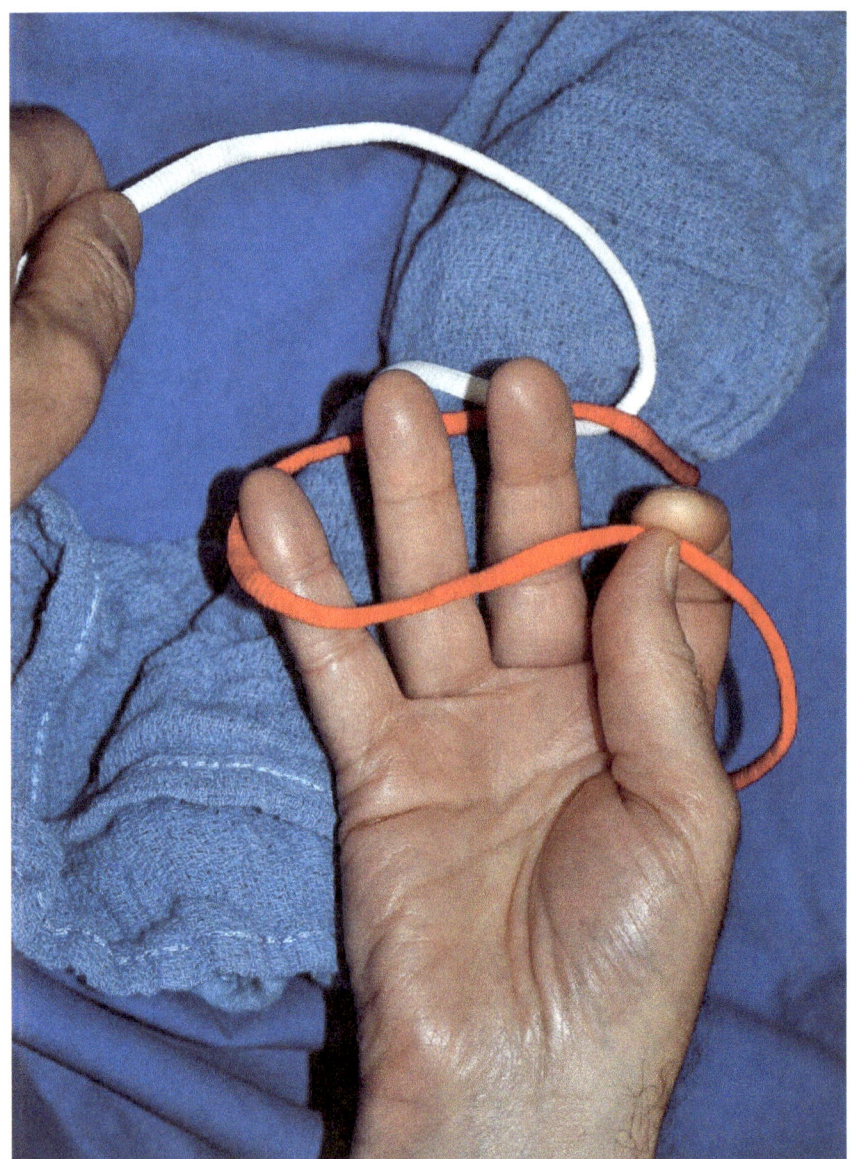

Figure 61.

Step 12. Supinate the right wrist with the red end along the back of the right fingers. This will wrap the short red end over the front of the middle, ring, and little fingers.

PLACING SUTURES & KNOT TYING

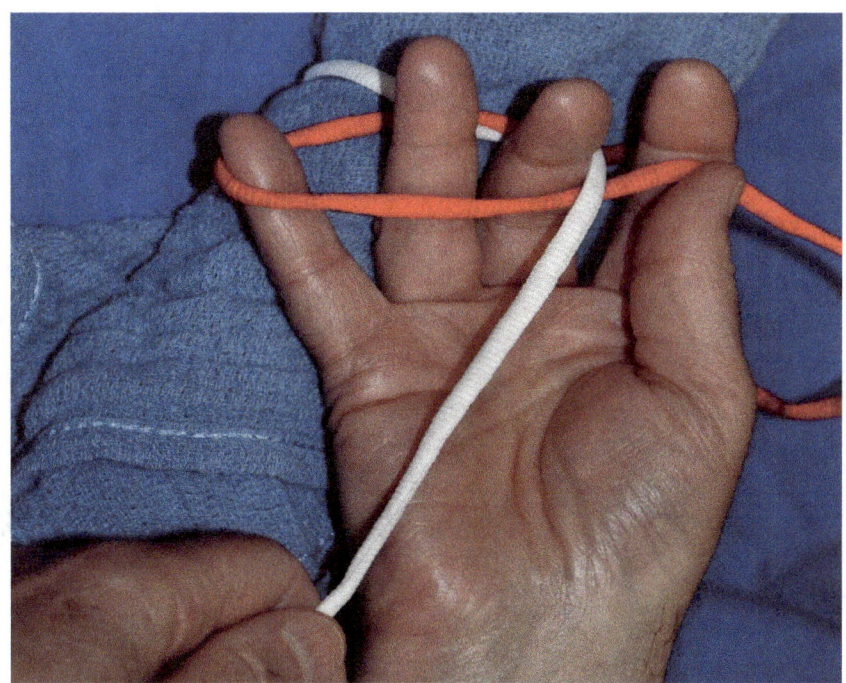

Figure 62.
Step 13. Cross the long white end over the red end.

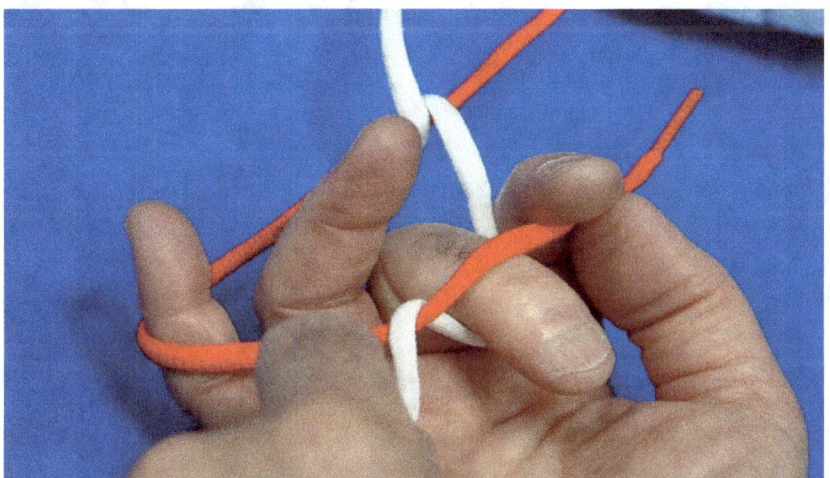

Figure 63.
Step 14. Now curl the right middle finger over the long white end held by the left hand, and under the short red end, held by the right hand.

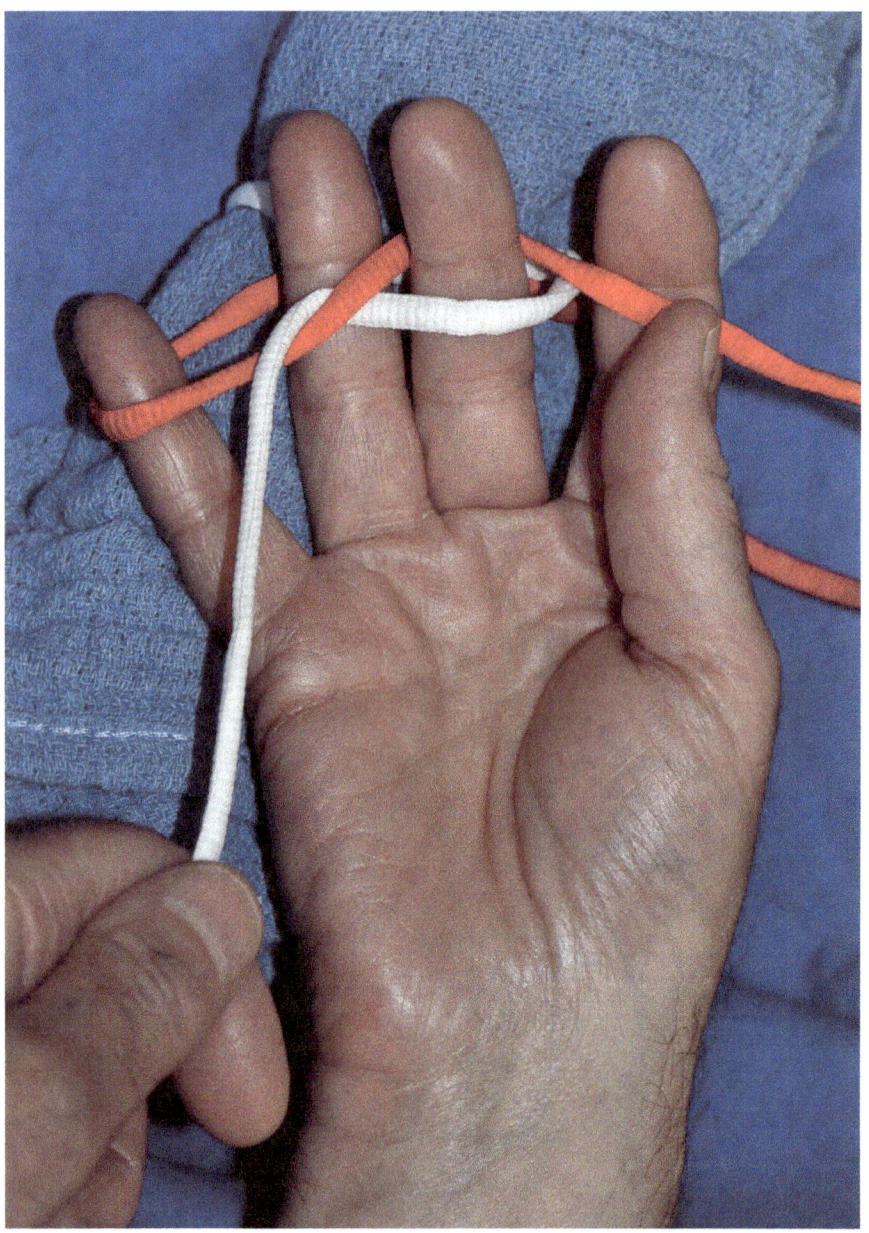

Figure 64.
Step 15. Straighten the middle finger to bring the red end over the long white end in a clockwise direction.

PLACING SUTURES & KNOT TYING

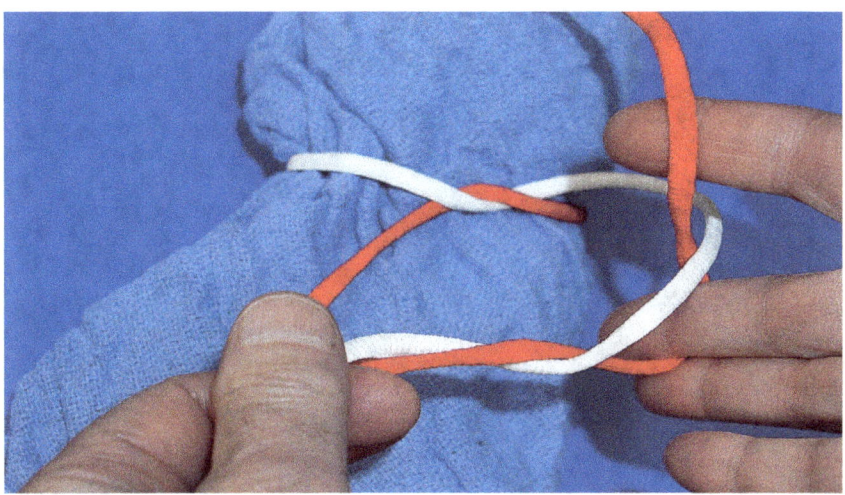

Figure 65.
Step 16. Pronate the right wrist at the same time as bringing the red loop on the back of the middle finger over the long white end.

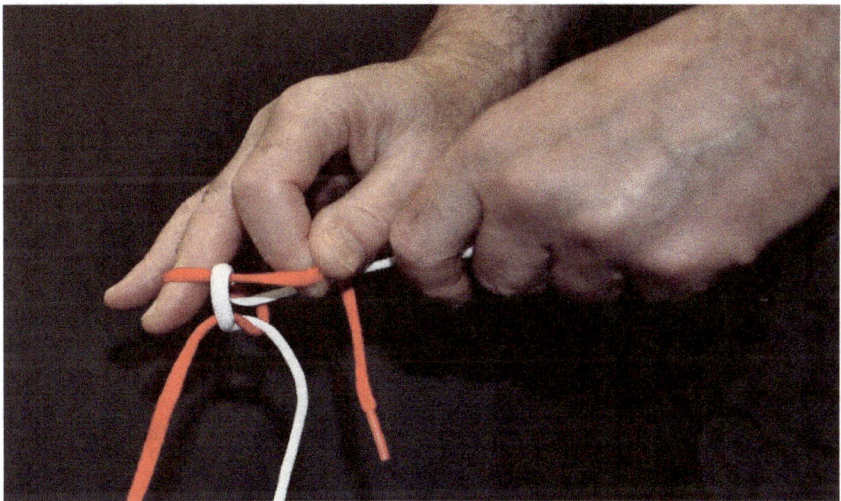

Figure 66.
Step 17. Continue to extend the middle finger of the right hand whilst pronating the right wrist. This will pull the short end under the longer white end. Release the short red end from between the right thumb and index. Continue to pull your right hand away from the knot, pulling red loop on the back of right middle finger until the short red end has come completely through the loop formed by the long white end.

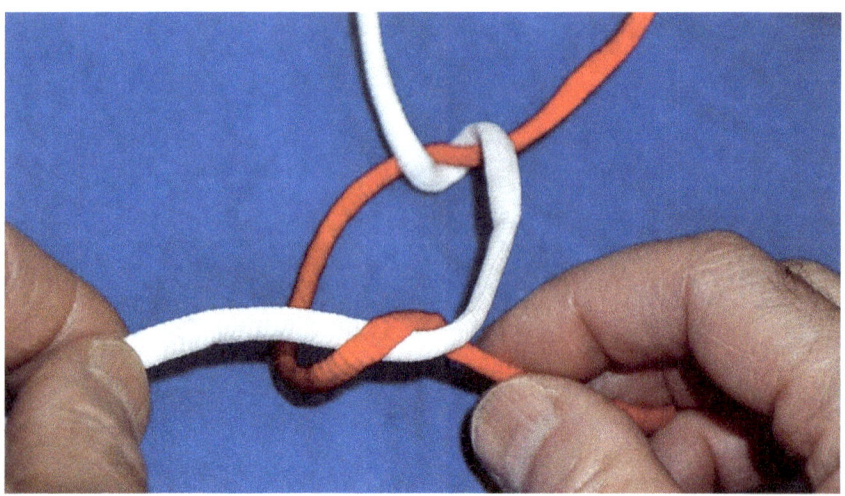

Figure 67.
Step 18. Grasp the short end with the thumb and index finger of the right hand. Using both hands simultaneously, pull each end, tightening the second throw onto the first knot. For the purposes of this illustration, the first knot has not been tightened down. Normally it would be snug against the skin. See Figure 70.

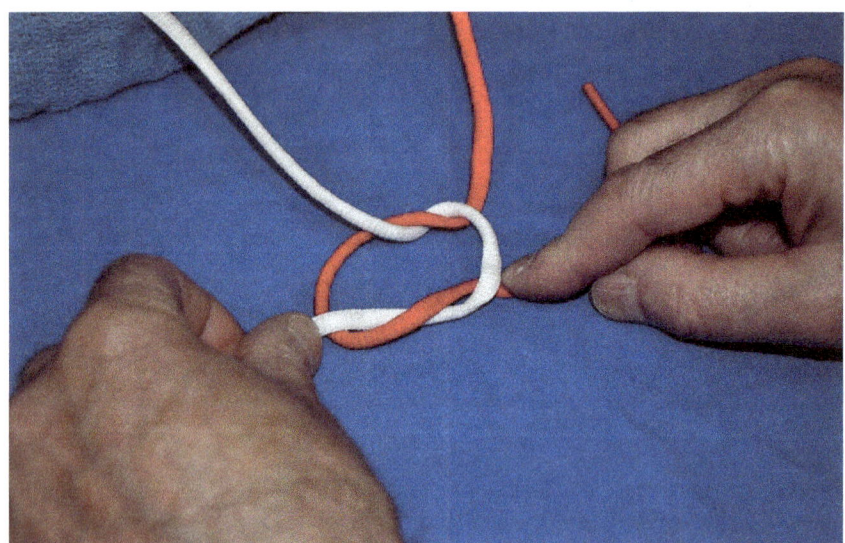

Figure 68.
Step 19. Further tightening of the knot.

PLACING SUTURES & KNOT TYING

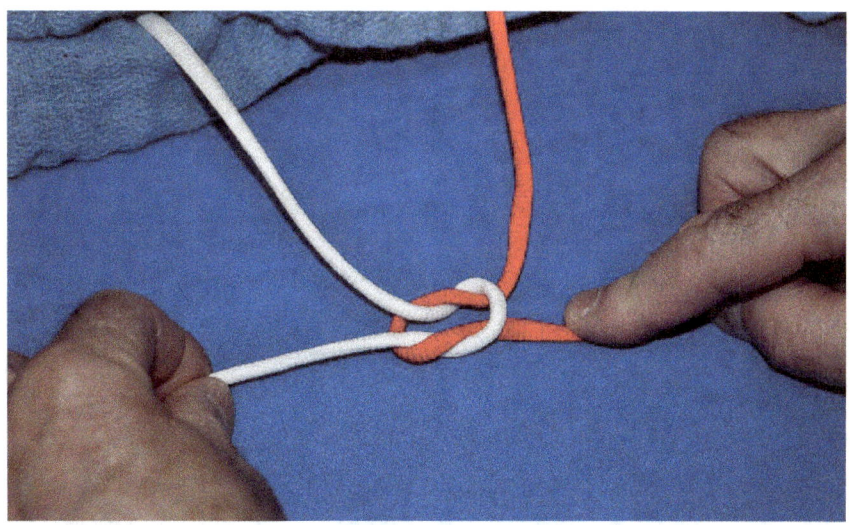

Figure 69.
Step 20. Tightening down a double square knot.

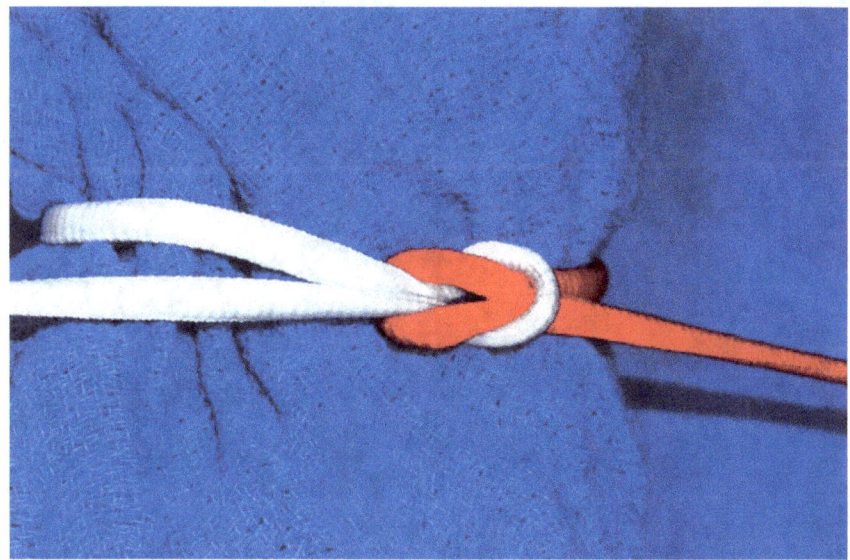

Figure 70.
Step 21. Both throws of a square knot tightened down snugly against the tissue.

b. Two-handed knot

A two-handed knot may be used to place a surgeon's knot when tying drains.

Step 1 is identical to a one-handed knot (Figure 49).

For a clockwise turn, begin with the index finger, crossing the long end in front of the short end. For a counterclockwise turn begin with the thumb crossing the long end behind the short end.

Here are the steps for a clockwise turn.

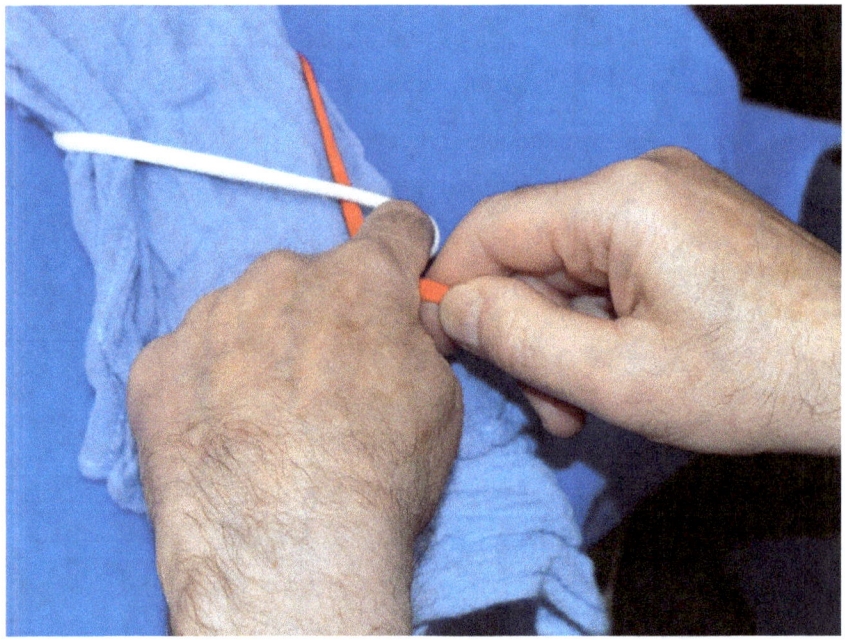

Figure 71.
Step 2. Pronate the left wrist so that the long white end is now curled over the outside of the left index finger, passing the long white end across and in front of the short red end.

PLACING SUTURES & KNOT TYING

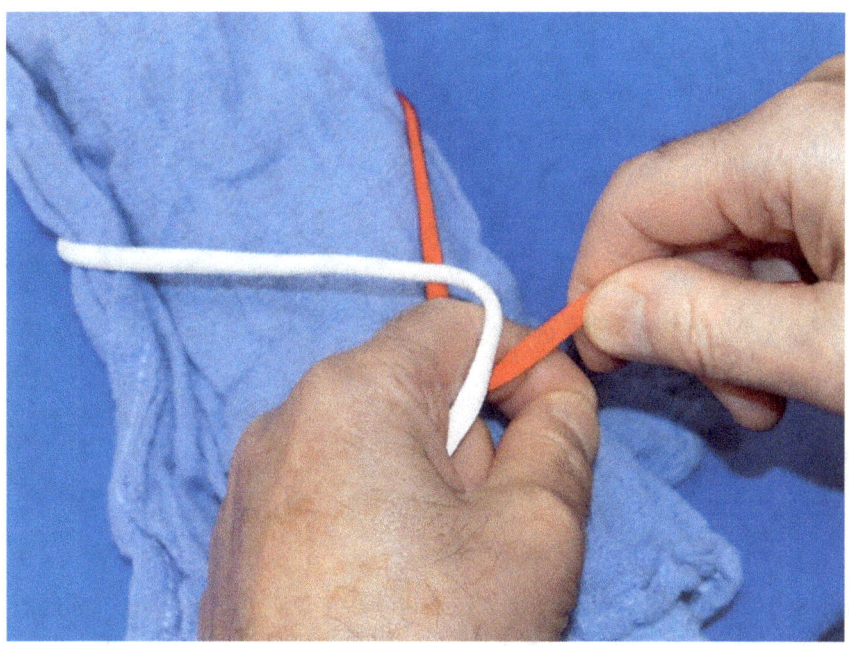

Figure 72.
Step 3. Place your index finger and thumb together behind the short end.

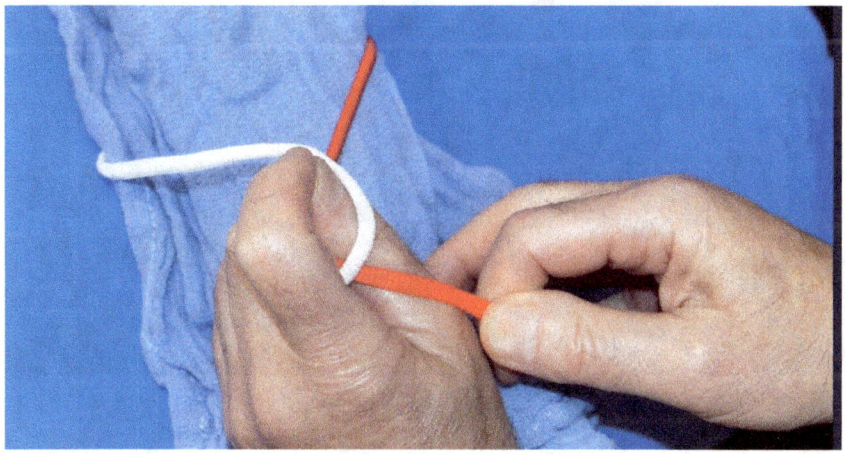

Figure 73.
Step 4. Extend the left wrist and bring the thumb and index finger together and forwards from behind, into the loop you have created,

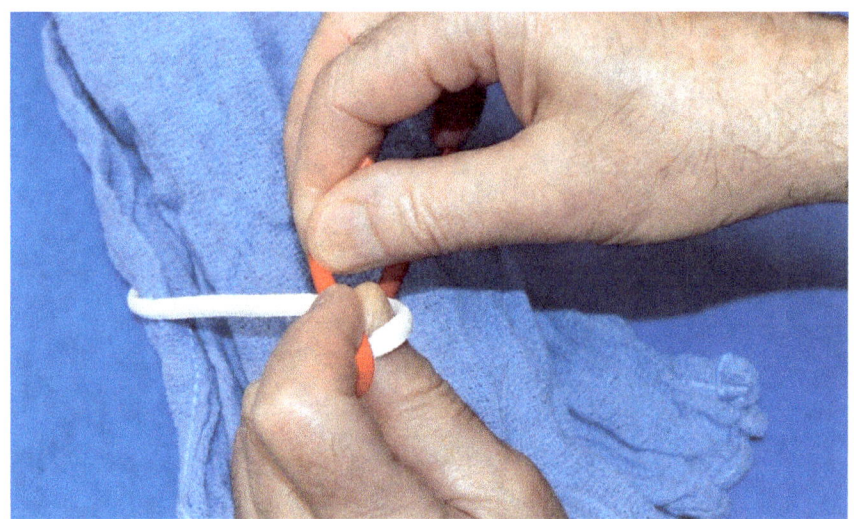

Figure 74.
Step 5. Using the right hand, cross the short end over the long white end into the cleft between the left index and thumb, which now grasps the short end.

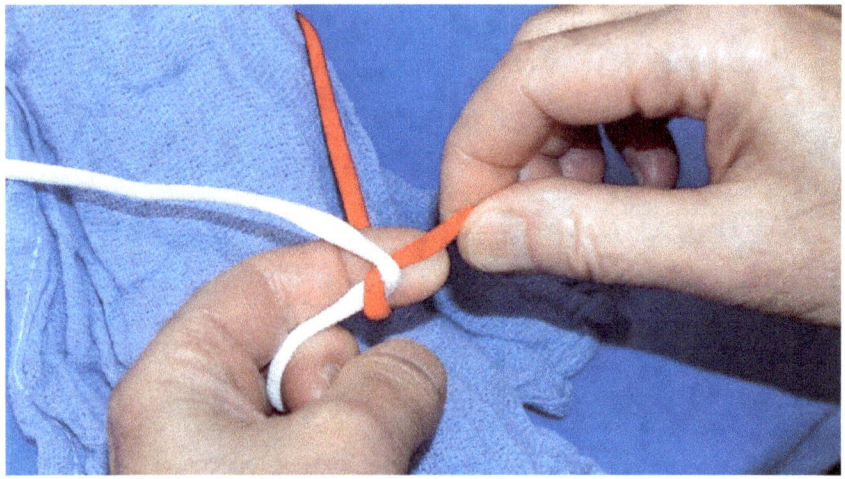

Figure 75.
Step 6. Now, release the short end from the right hand and using the left thumb and index, flex and supinate the left wrist bringing the short red end around and in front of the long white end. The short end is now under the long end, facing to the right. The right hand grasps the short end again. For a surgeon's knot, repeat steps 3,4,5, and 6 to create two throws in the same direction. Then proceed to **step 7.**

PLACING SUTURES & KNOT TYING

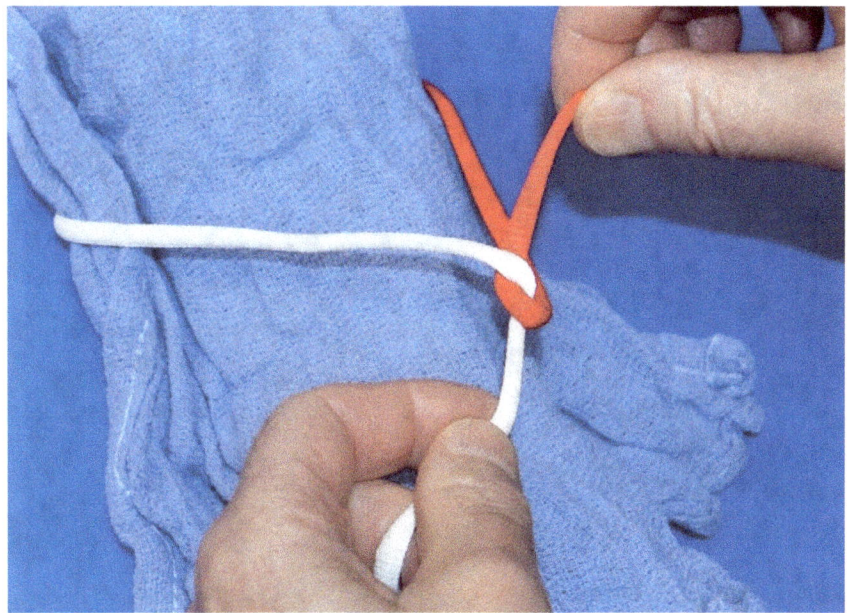

Figure 76.
Step 7. Pull on both ends simultaneously.

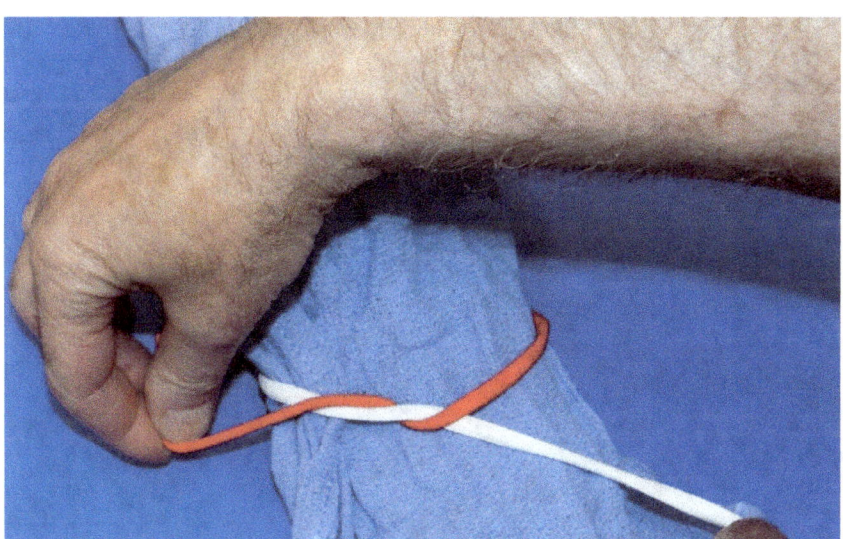

Figure 77.
Step 8. Cross the right hand in front of the left to make a square knot. Pull both ends simultaneously.

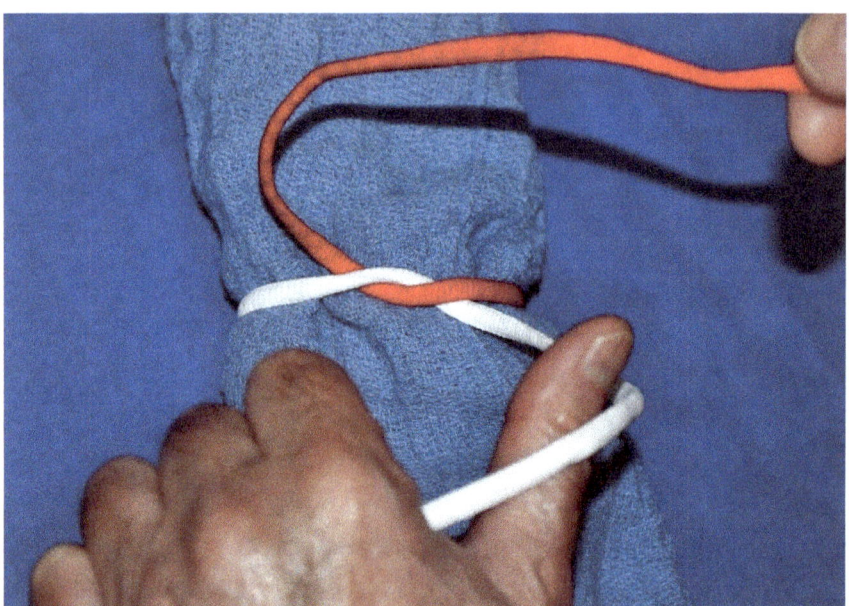

Figure 78.
Step 9. For the next counterclockwise throw, uncross the hands and curl the left thumb under long white end, which now rolls around the outer side of the thumb.

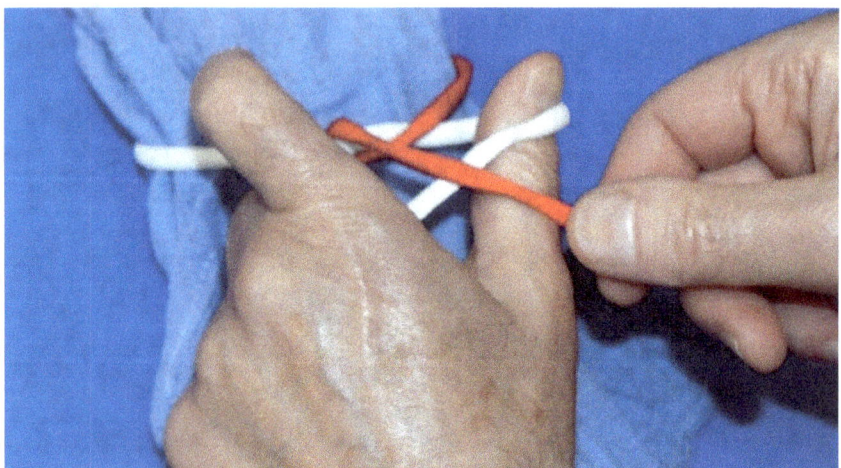

Figure 79.
Step 10. Cross the short red end over the left thumb using the right hand.

PLACING SUTURES & KNOT TYING

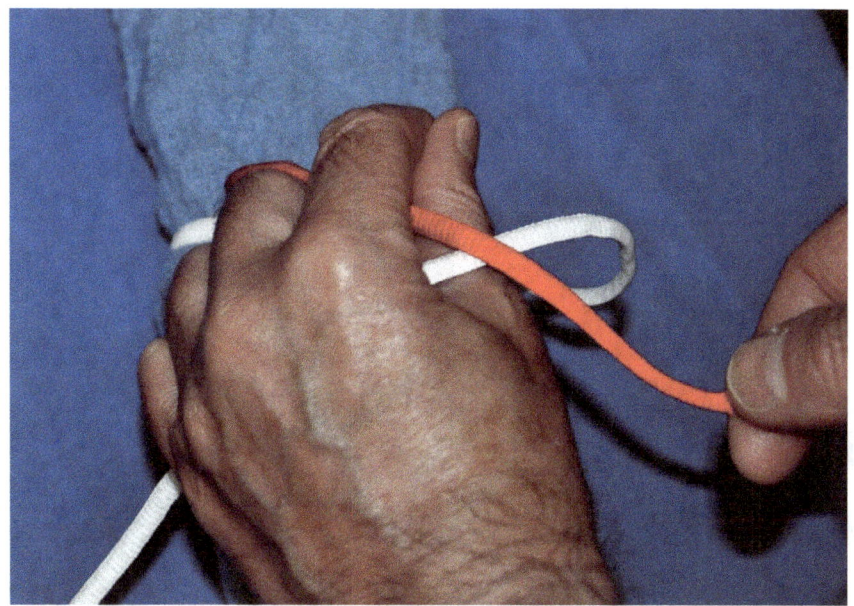

Figure 80.
Step 11. Pinch the left thumb and index together.

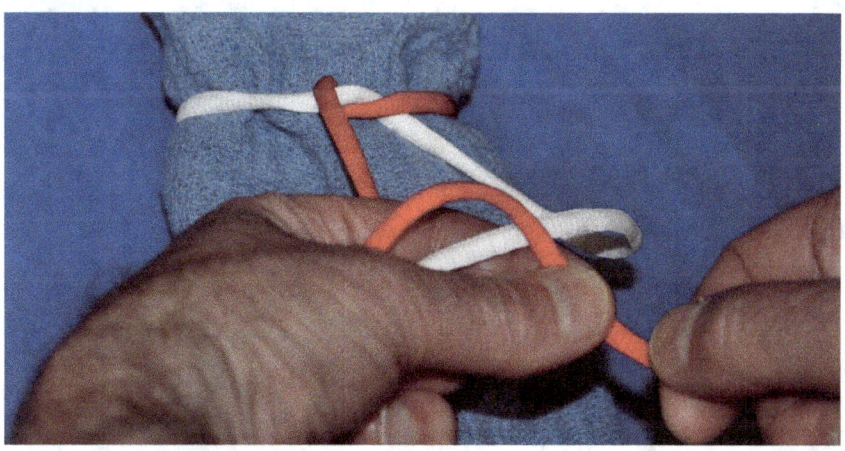

Figure 81.
Step 12. Curl the thumb and index around behind the long white end whilst flexing and supinating the left wrist and grasp the short red end.

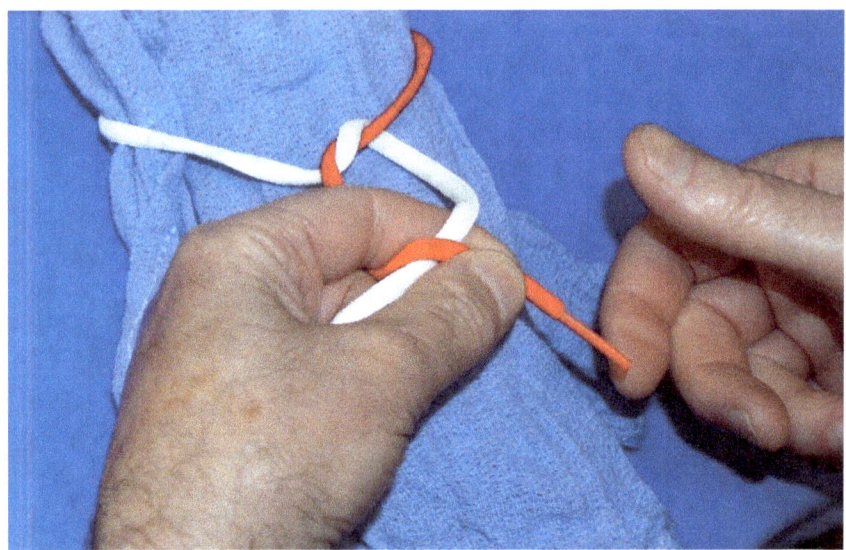

Figure 82.
Step 13. Release the short red end from your right hand.

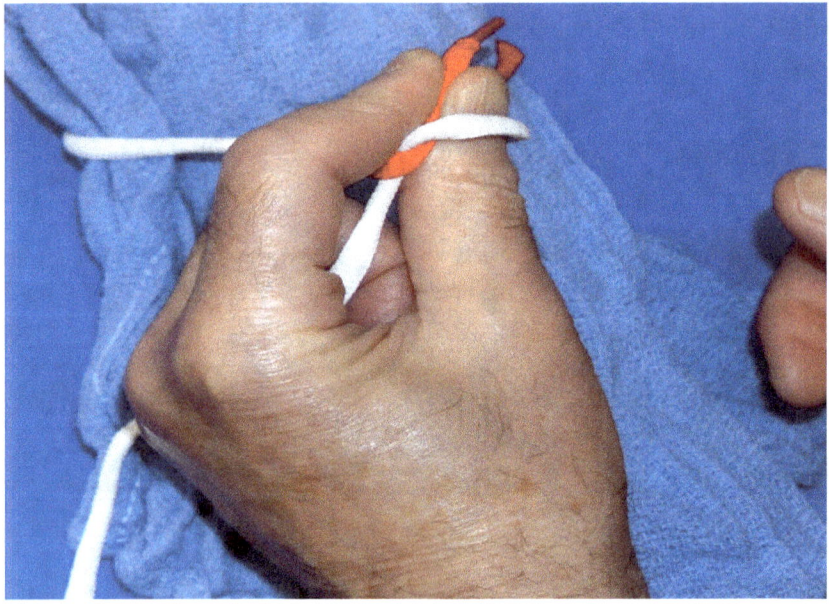

Figure 83.
Step 14. Extend the left wrist, bringing the short red end through the loop and under the long white end.

PLACING SUTURES & KNOT TYING

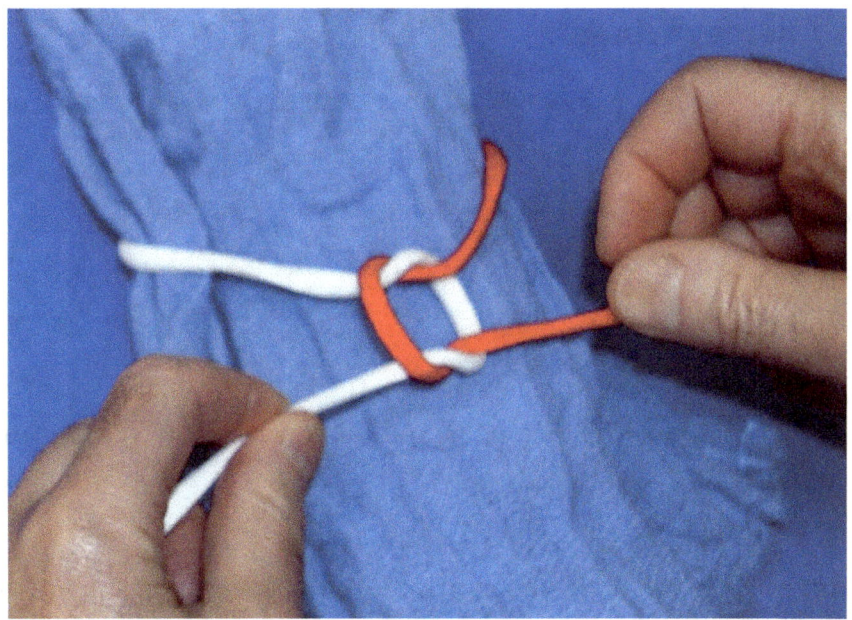

Figure 84

Step 15. Grasp the short end with the right hand and pull both ends simultaneously, tightening the second loop down to fit snugly against the first.

For an initial counterclockwise turn, reverse the steps starting with a counterclockwise maneuver, as in **Step 9** (Figure 78).

c. Aberdeen Knot

A useful technique to finish a subcuticular suture is the Aberdeen knot.

This technique buries the knot.

Stage I. Make a loop (loop one) from last bite in the closure. (Figure 85).

Stage II. Holding the needle end with the left hand (exiting right in Figure 85), grasp the long end, creating a second loop (loop two) and pull it through loop one that you created in Stage I. (Figure 86).

Stage III. Tighten loop one with index, ring, and middle fingers of right hand by pulling on loop two that you pulled through loop one whilst maintaining the tension on the needle end of the suture. (Figure 86).

Repeat Stages I, II and III.

Stage IV. Now place the needle through the loop two held by the right hand and pull the needle end so that the loop is cinched down. (Figures 87 and 88).

Stage V. Pass the needle through the wound to the skin surface on either side of the wound and cut suture at skin level (Figure 89).

PLACING SUTURES & KNOT TYING

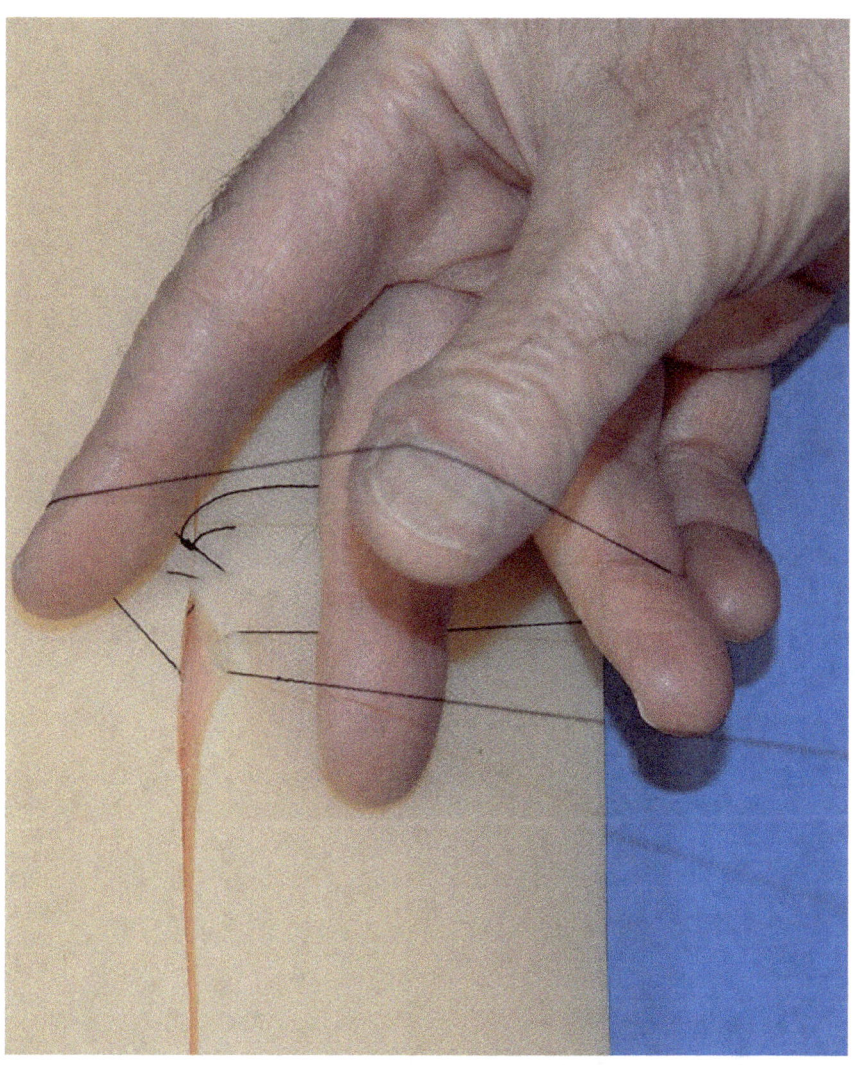

Figure 85.
Stage I and II. Making a loop from the previous stitch with your right hand (loop one) Pull long (needle) end partially through the loop with the thumb and middle finger of the right hand creating second loop (loop two).

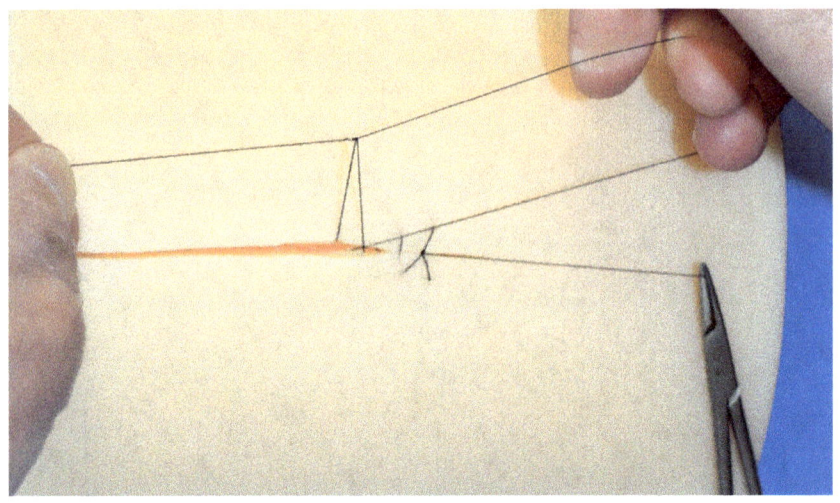

Figures 86.

Stage III. Pulling loop two, tightening with right hand on right, whilst keeping long needle end of suture taught in left hand. Repeat **Stages I, II and III** two times.

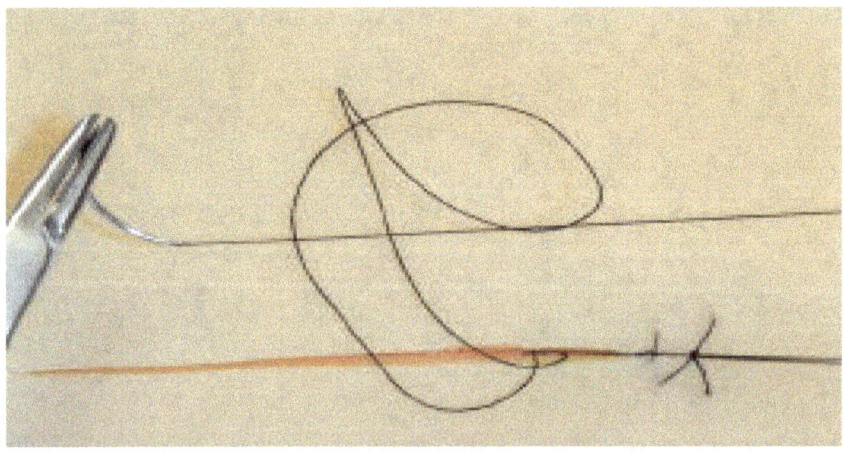

Figure 87

Stage IV. Now place needle end through loop two and pull needle end until loop is snug.

PLACING SUTURES & KNOT TYING

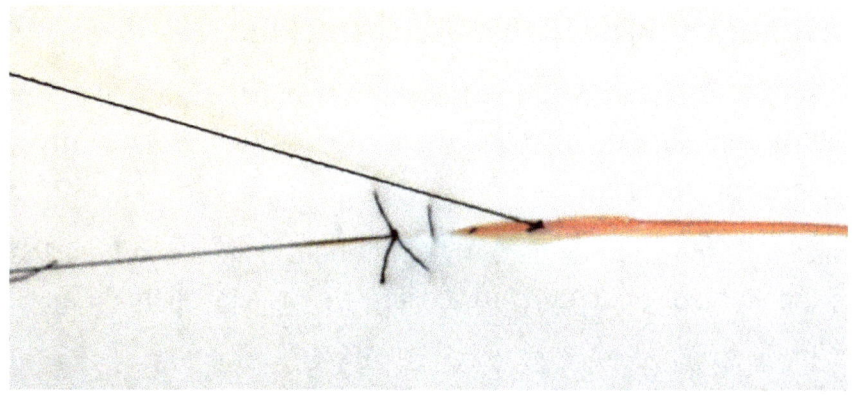

Figure 88.
Stage IV. Place needle through loop and pull needle down tight until loop is snug.

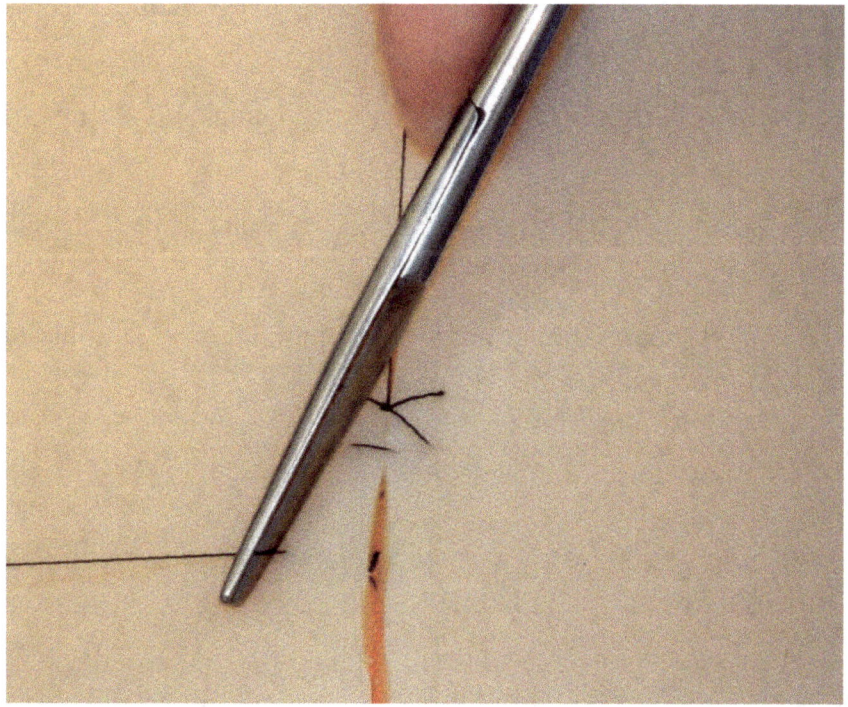

Figure 89.
Stage V. Pass needle from inside the wound through the skin and cut the suture at skin level as shown.

d. Withdrawing a stitch or 'backtracking.'

If for any reason, such as a bad suture 'bite' or 'button-holing' the skin in a running subcuticular stitch, you must withdraw a stitch, this is surprisingly easy.

Stage I. Grasp the needle with the needle holder and hold the proximal end of the suture on tension with the left hand. (Figure 90).

Stage II. Pull the proximal suture gently and direct the suage end of the needle back into its exit hole. The suture will slide back through the tunnel. (Figures 91A and 91B).

Stage III. Grasp the needle with the needle holder on the proximal side, withdrawing the needle (not shown).

Now you are ready to start your stitch again in a forward direction.

If you 'buttonholed' the skin with a subcuticular stitch, it would take two separate steps to reverse this.

- First loosen the suture loop on the skin side so that you can grasp the suture loop.
- Withdraw the needle to the skin side as above.
- Repeat again, withdrawing the needle back into the wound.
- Now you are ready to restart your stitch again in a forward direction.

PLACING SUTURES & KNOT TYING

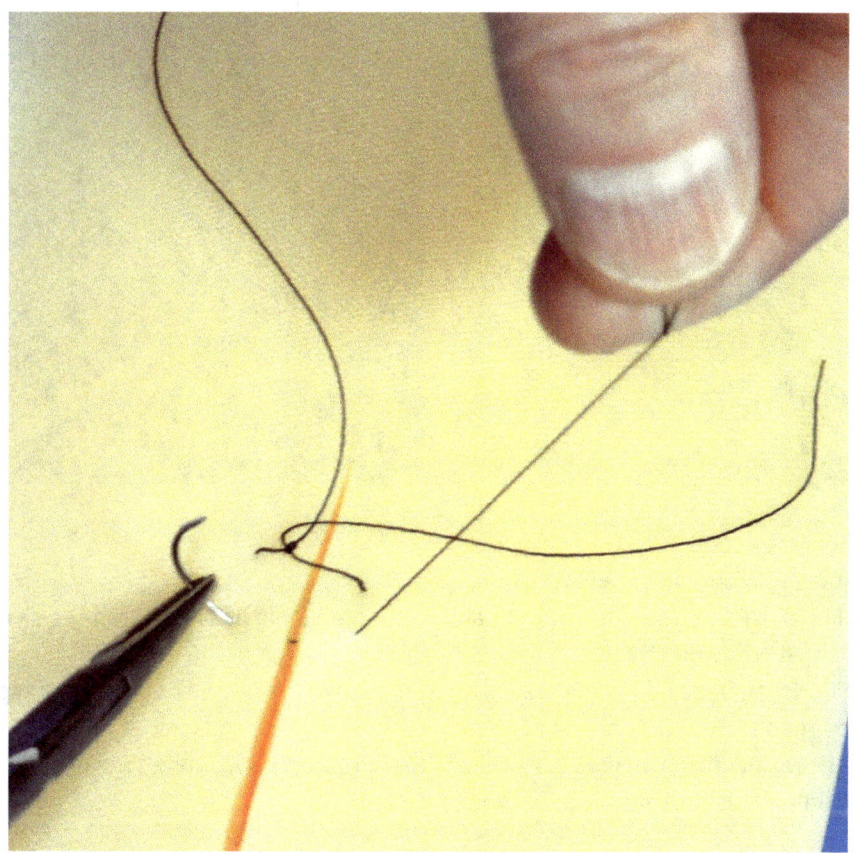

Figure 90.
Stage I. Withdrawing a suture bite:
Push the suage end of the needle back into the exit hole whilst applying constant tension to the proximal suture with the left hand.

KIRWAN'S OPERATION ROOM TECHNIQUES

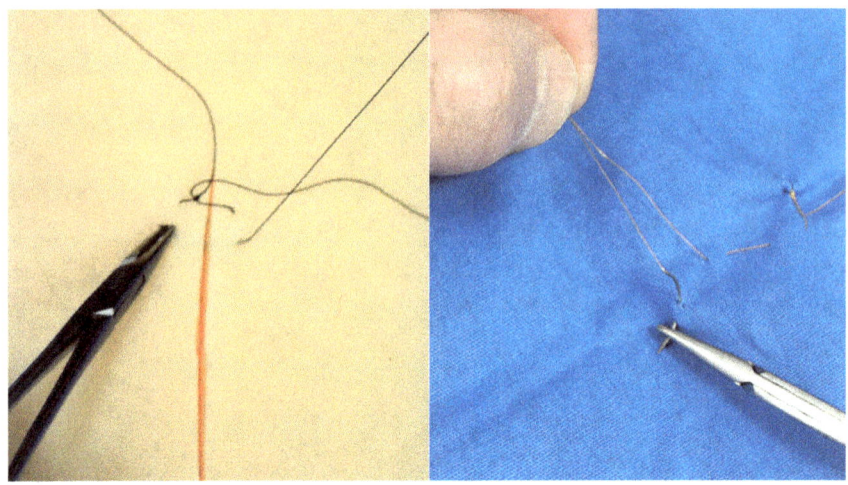

Figure 91A. and 91B.
Stage II. Withdrawing a suture bite:
91A (left). Pull back with the left hand once the needle has reentered the skin along its previous track.
91B (right). Once it is at the stage, you can release the needle holder and grasp the needle on the proximal side, withdrawing the needle. If you have 'buttonhole' the skin, you will have to repeat this maneuver one time until the needle eye is presenting in the wound.

SUTURE CUTTING

06

A suture should be presented in profile for cutting.

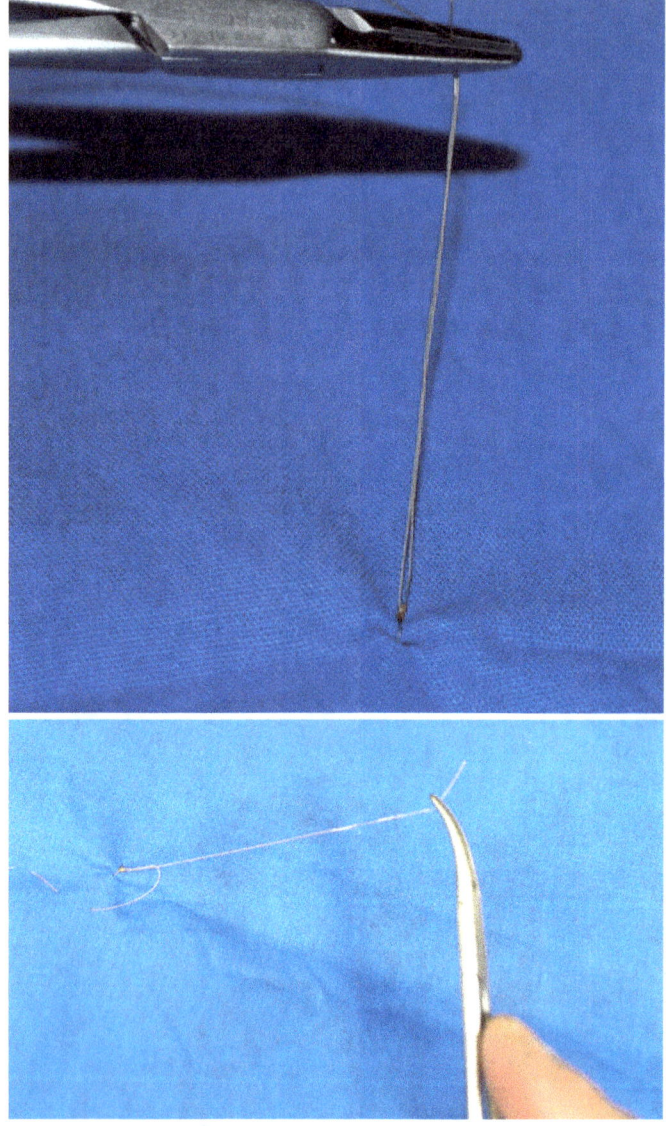

Figure 92.
Present the suture away from the assistant, in profile, so that they can clearly see to cut, *not end-on* as shown in Figure 93 below.

SUTURE CUTTING

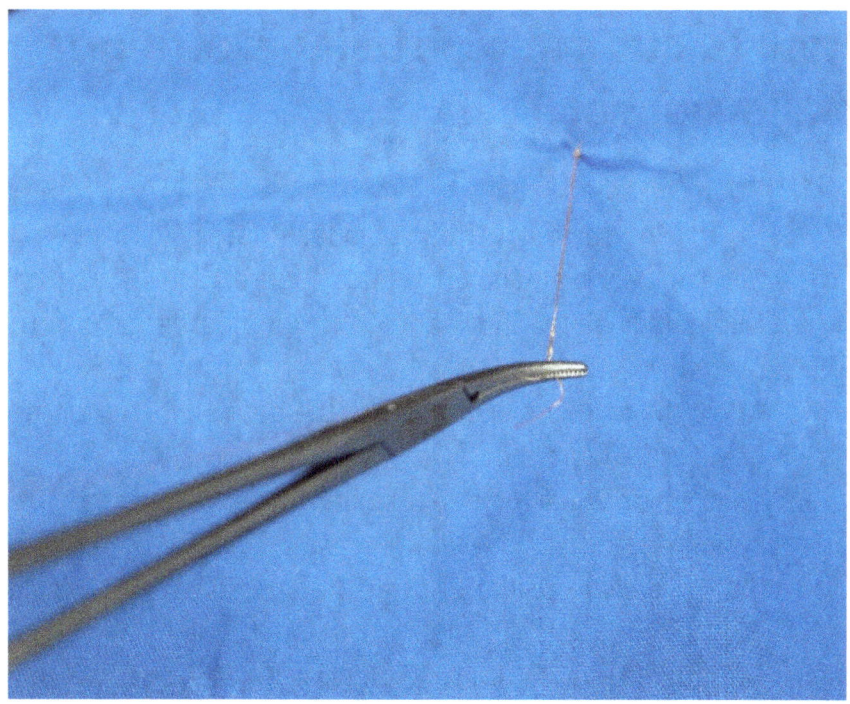

Figure 93.
Do not hold the suture towards the assistant, as this prevents the assistant from being able to view the suture to cut.

How to cut a suture using a straight Mayo scissor.

1. Open scissor blades.
2. Bow string suture over back blade. Figure 94.
3. Slide scissor blade down to knot. Figure 95
4. Supinate wrist at an angle of 45 degrees from full pronation.
5. Angle the scissors according to the desired length of tails of suture. Figure 95.
6. Tails are one quarter inch for skin suture, unless otherwise specified.
7. Tails are close to the knot at the start of a subcuticular suture.
8. Do not cut on the knot. Feel with the scissor and then angle the blades.
9. **CUT!!** Cutting is one action, do not hesitate.
10. Do not rotate your wrist as you cut. Supinate, then cut.
11. Cut both suture threads at the same time, *Otherwise, the knot will pull through and loosen!*
12. Do not turn your wrist away from you, i.e., do not pronate!
13. You should be able to cut a suture by feel, without looking at it. Sometimes you will not be able to see the knot.
14. Cut sutures using the ends of the scissor blades.
15. If using a hemostat to apply traction to a suture or to prevent it being "pulled through" use the tips of the jaws. Figure 92.
16. If necessary, cut the end of the suture, leaving the hemostat attached to the suture. Figure 96.

SUTURE CUTTING

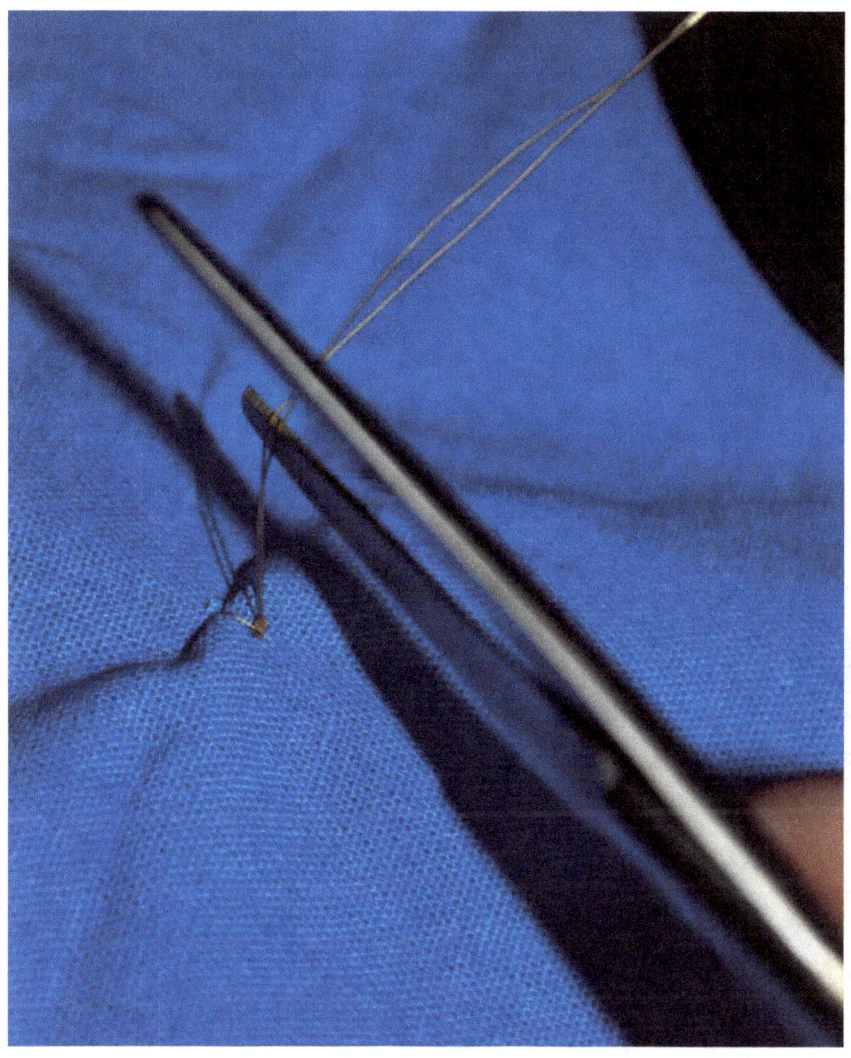

Figure 94.
Bow string suture over the blade furthest from you. Keep the blades open!

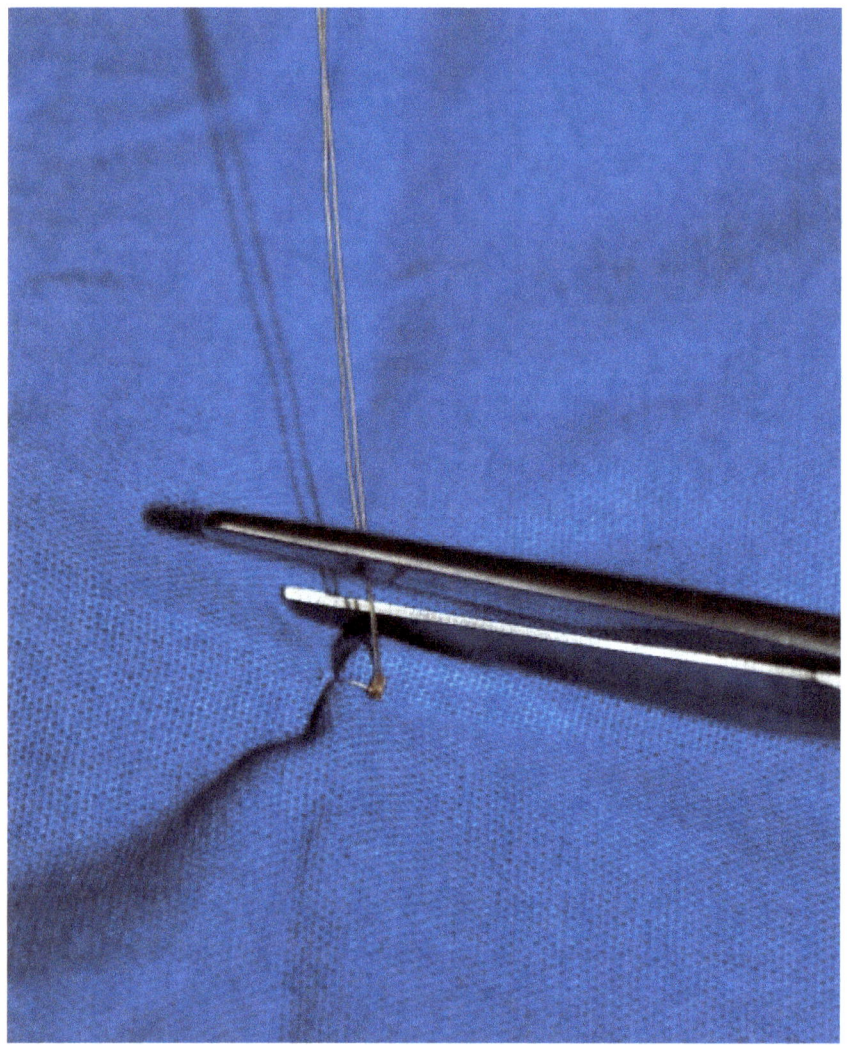

Figure 95.
Angle the scissors according to the desired length of the suture tails.

SUTURE CUTTING

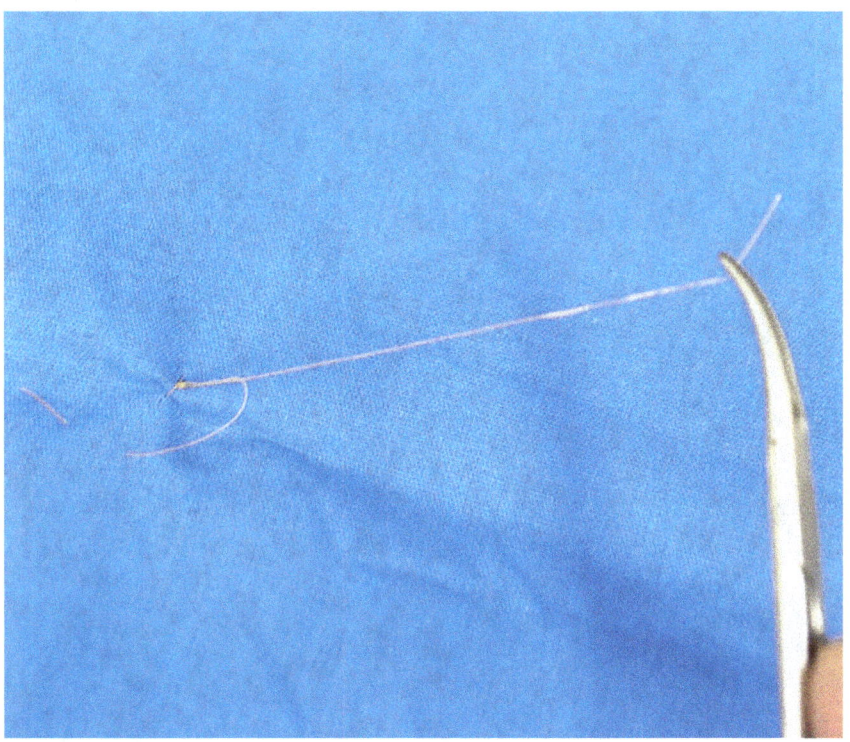

Figure 96.
If you are grasping a suture to apply tension to it or to present it for cutting, grasp the suture using the tip of hemostat jaws. Cut beyond the hemostat if the hemostat is to remain attached.

CLOSING WITH STERISTRIPS

07

Steristrips can be used instead of a final subcuticular suture or in addition to one. They should be placed at ninety degrees to the incisions and there should be a space between successive strips to allow blood to escape from the incision into the overlying dressing. The size of the Steristrips will vary depending on the location. Half inch for body, quarter inch for face and small incisions and one eighth inch for eyelids. Steristrips may also be used to hold down and secure both ends of a non-absorbable Nylon or Prolene subcuticular suture.

Cut the Steristrips 1/3 length and remove the end strip. The assistant holds the Steristrips at each upper corner with the sticky side towards the assistant.

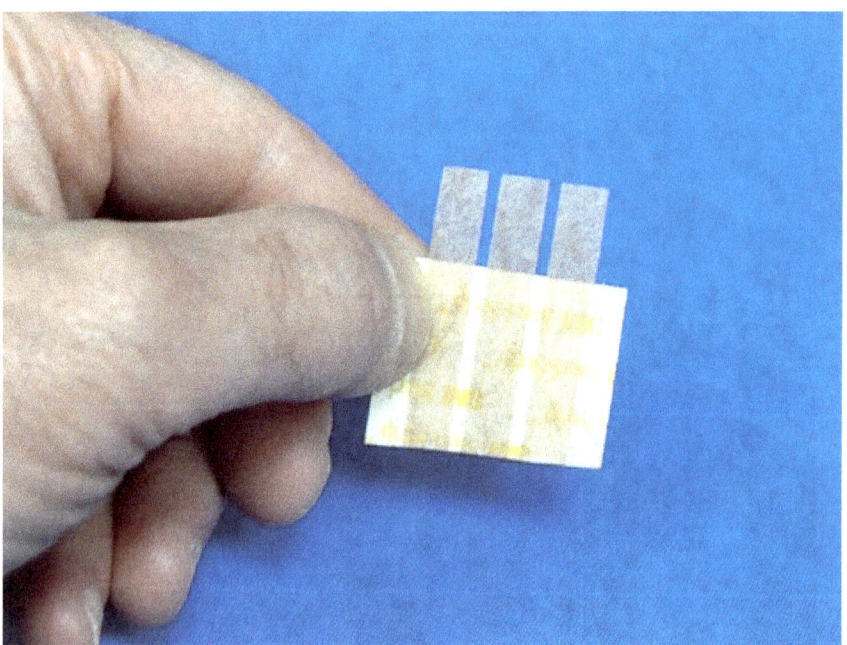

Figure 97.
Cut Steristrips in thirds. Hold the sticky side up and toward the assistant. Hold both upper corners with thumb and index finger, not single-handed as shown in Figure 97.

CLOSING WITH STERISTRIPS

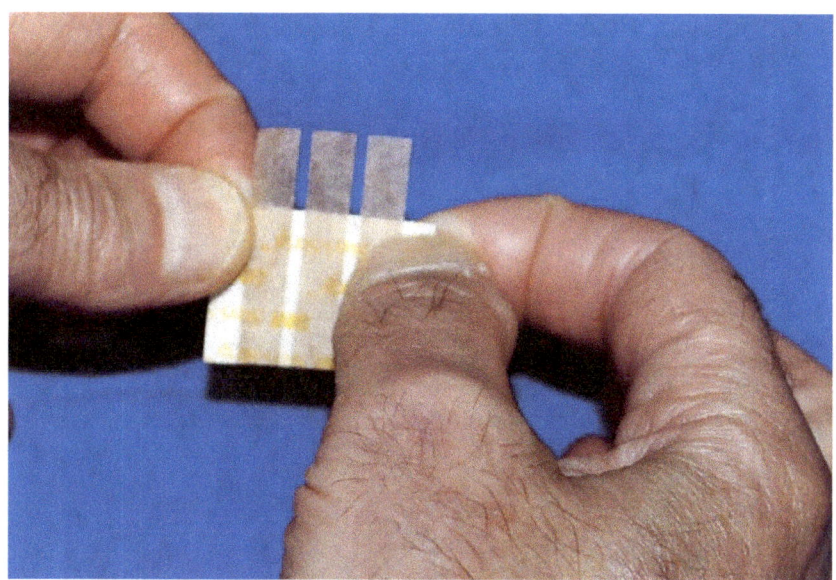

Figure 98.
Pictured is incorrect presentation of Steristrips, holding both top corners with sticky side facing surgeon.

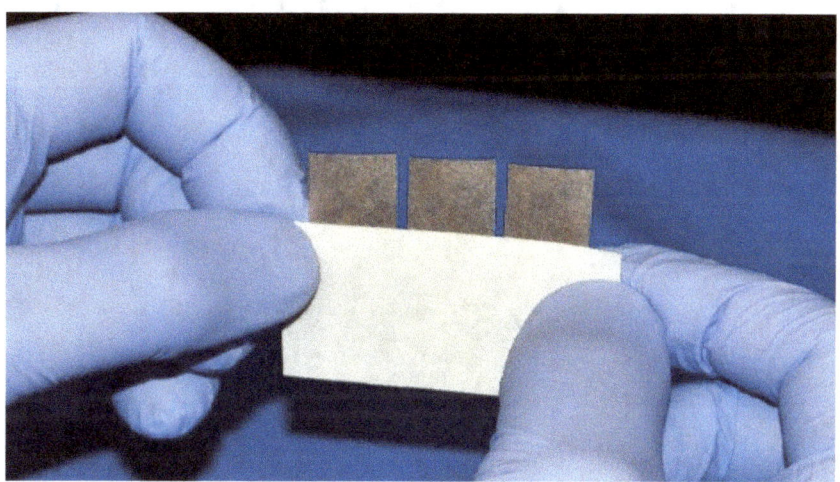

Figure 99.
Pictured is correct presentation of Steristrips. Assistant's view, holding both top corners. Steristrips should face surgeon with sticky side towards the assistant

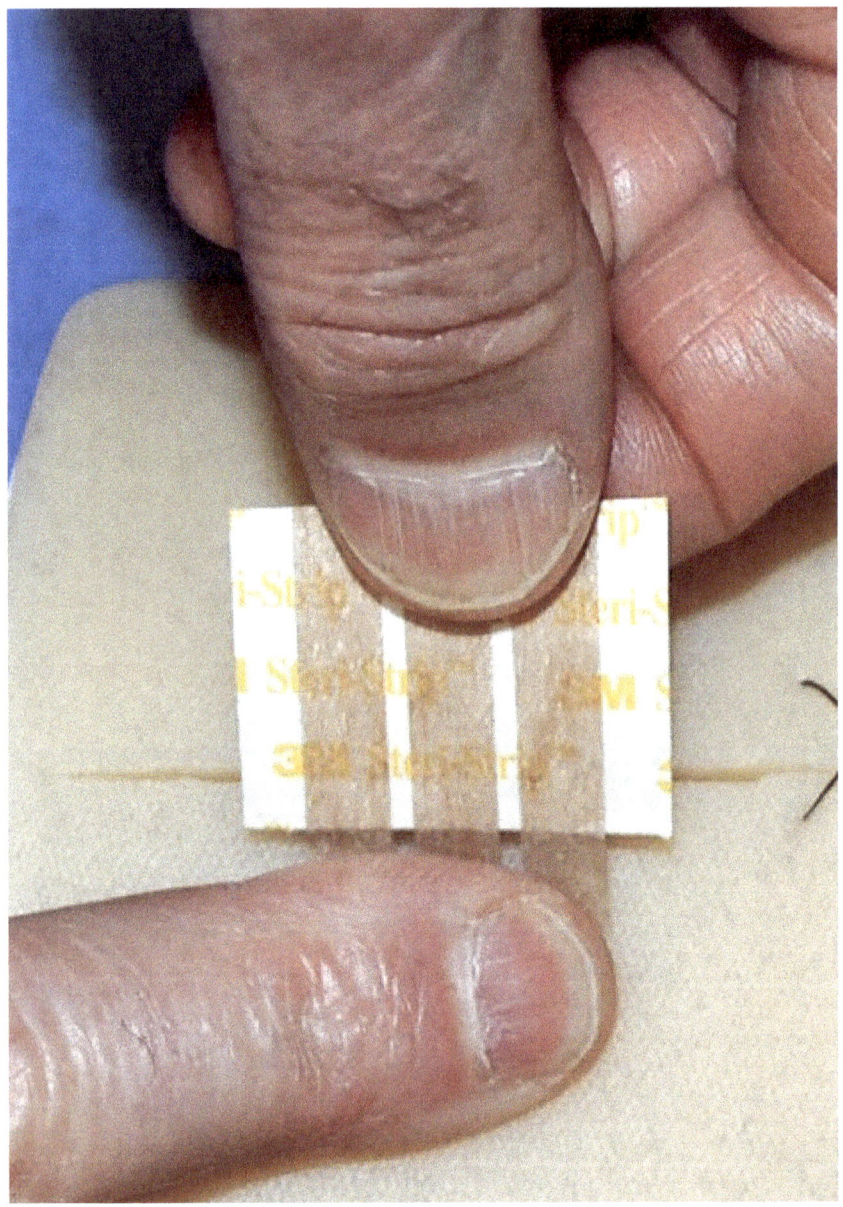

Figure 100.
Apply Steristrips in groups of three. Press down on one side of the incision, pushing the incision closed. Peel off the paper backing, laying down the Steristrips on the other side of the incision.

CLOSING WITH STERISTRIPS

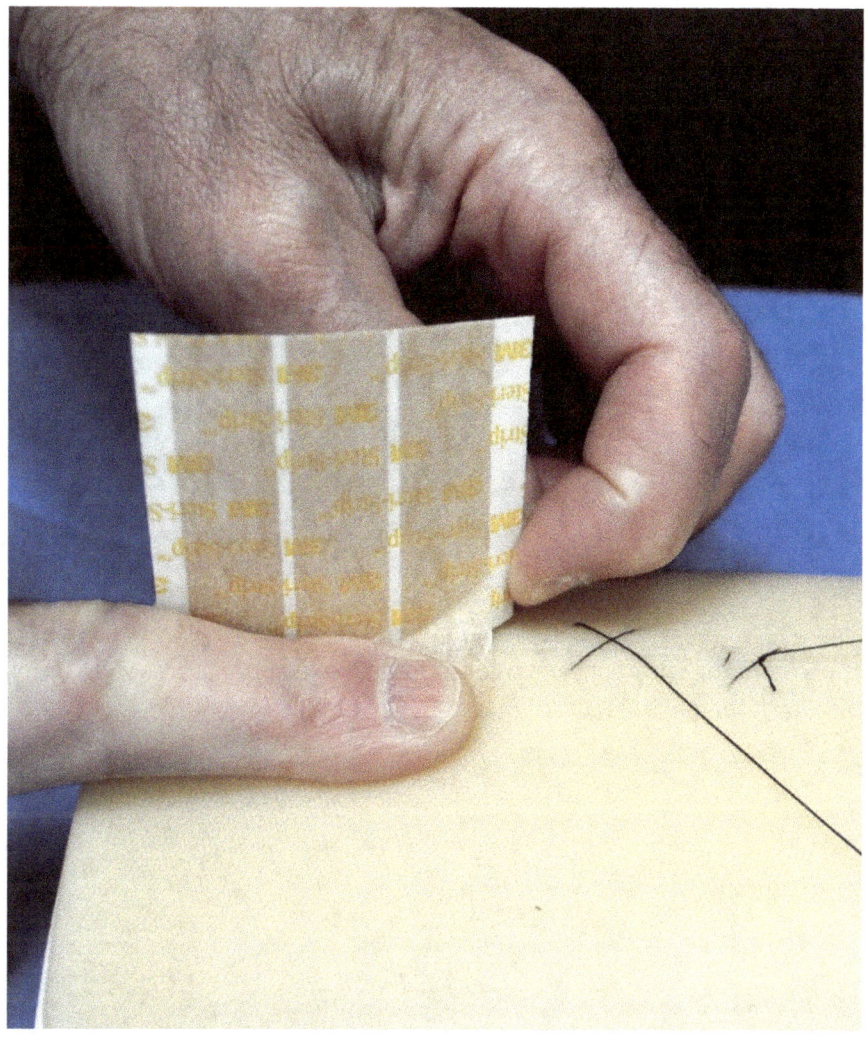

Figure 101.
Apply ½" Steristrips in groups of three. Press down on one side of the incision pushing the incision closed. Peel the paper backing away, starting with the corner closest to the wound. Continue to lay the Steristrips down on the other side of the incision.

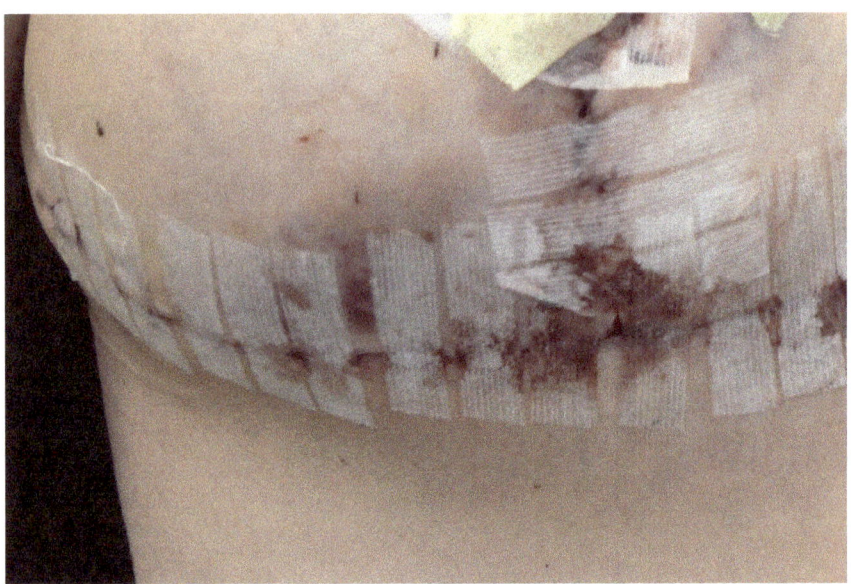

Figure 102.
Apply Steristrips in groups of three. Pictured is example of a breast reduction case, postoperative view.

PASSING INSTRUMENTS

08

Passing instruments must be a seamless process and should not necessitate the surgeon turning their head to see and retrieve an instrument, thereby interrupting their attention on the operative field. This would waste time and is inefficient. Therefore, it is important to pass instruments correctly. Place an instrument in the palm, not the fingers. If an instrument is placed on the fingers and not the palm, the surgeon is unable to grasp it and it will fall out of the hand.

Don't hesitate! It is preferable to mistakenly pass the wrong instrument and have the surgeon return it rather than hesitate to offer any instrument.

PASSING INSTRUMENTS

A. Passing a ring-handled instrument

Pass instruments to the surgeon by placing the handle of the instrument in the palm. **Here are some ways not to pass an instrument.** Absolutely avoid these maneuvers!

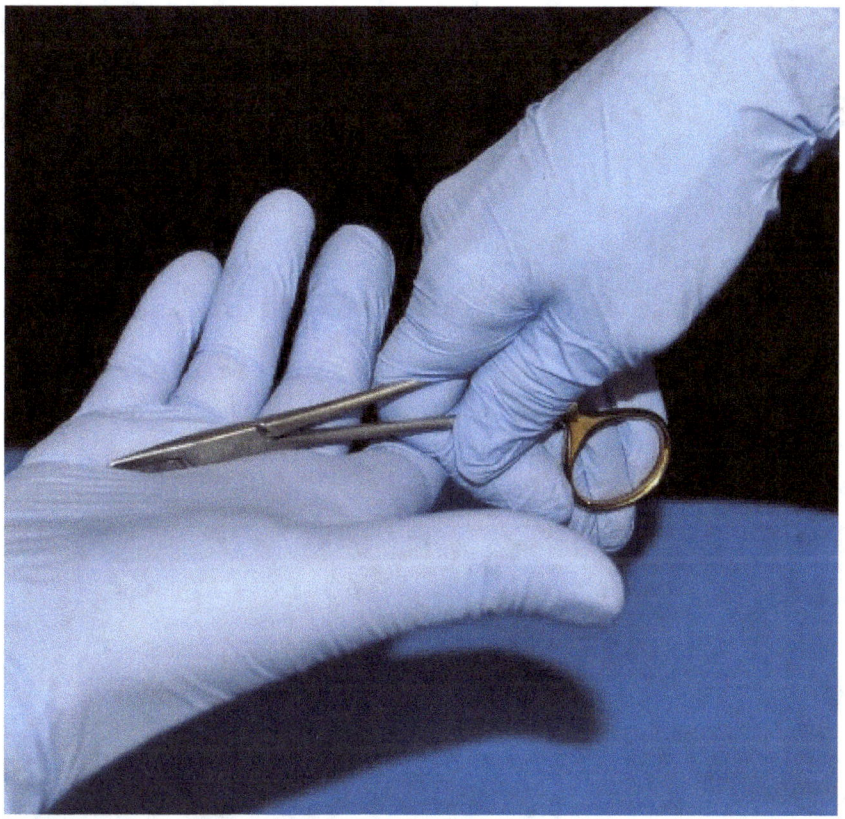

Figure 103.
Incorrect way to pass a ring-handled instrument. The handle, not the tip, should be placed in the surgeon's palm.

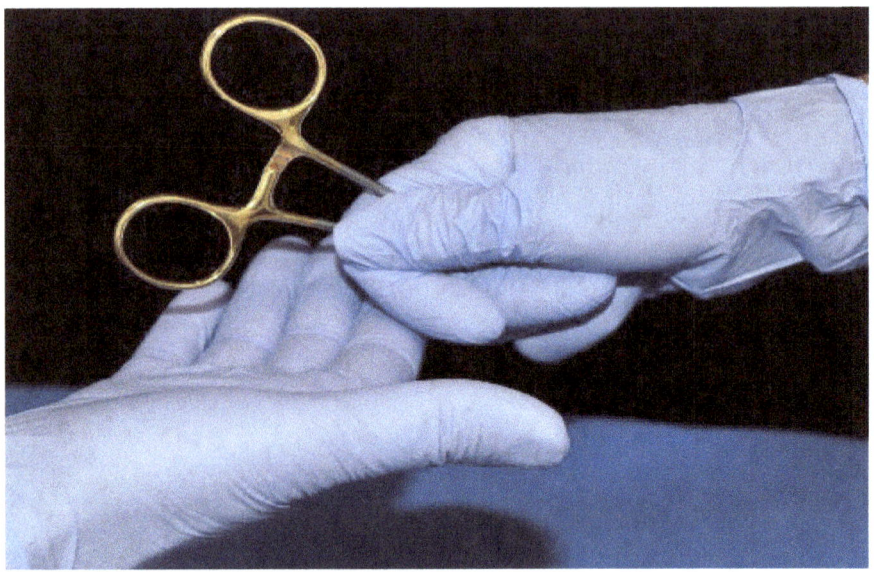

Figure 104.
Incorrect way to pass a ring-handled instrument. Surgeon must rotate instrument to use, which is unstable and may fall out of the palm. Surgeon's hand is on the left.

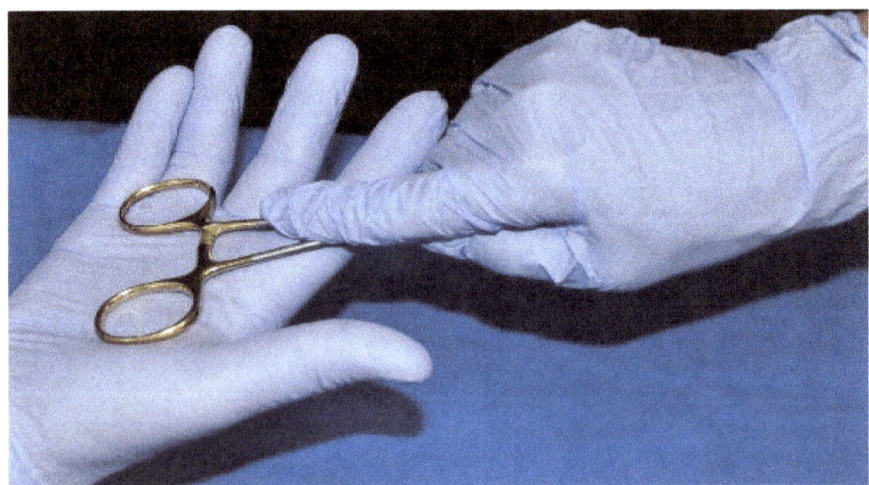

Figure 105.
Correct way to pass a ringed instrument to surgeon. The handle is placed firmly in the flat of the surgeon's **palm**. Surgeon's hand is on the left.

PASSING INSTRUMENTS

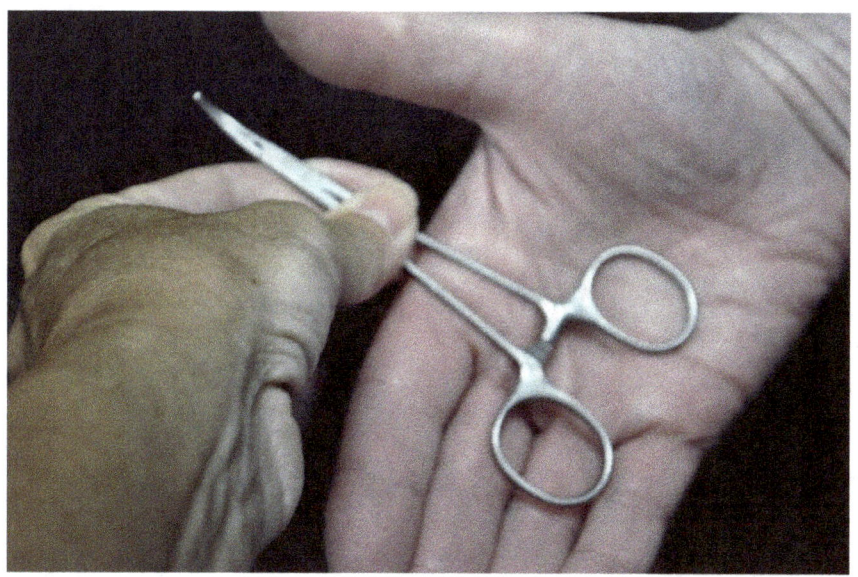

Figure 106.
Correct way to pass a hemostat. The points of the instrument face up and away from the palm of the surgeon. Surgeon's hand is on the right.

B. Holding and passing a knife

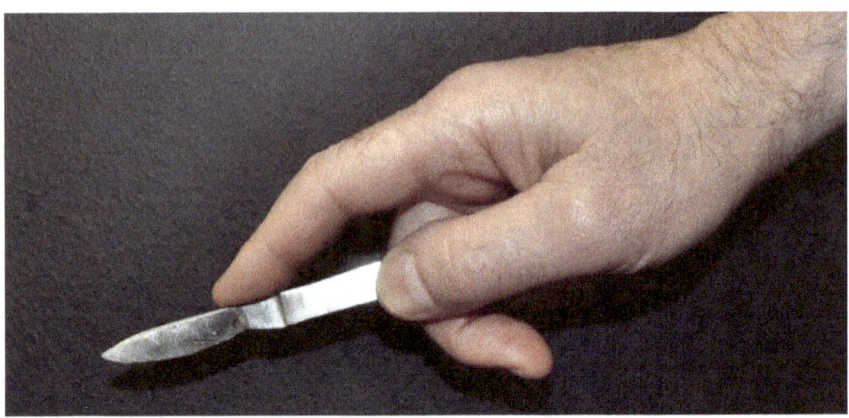

Figure 107.
Correct way to hold a knife in use. Index finger on back of handle close to and opposite blade edge. The knife handle is held between the thumb and middle finger.

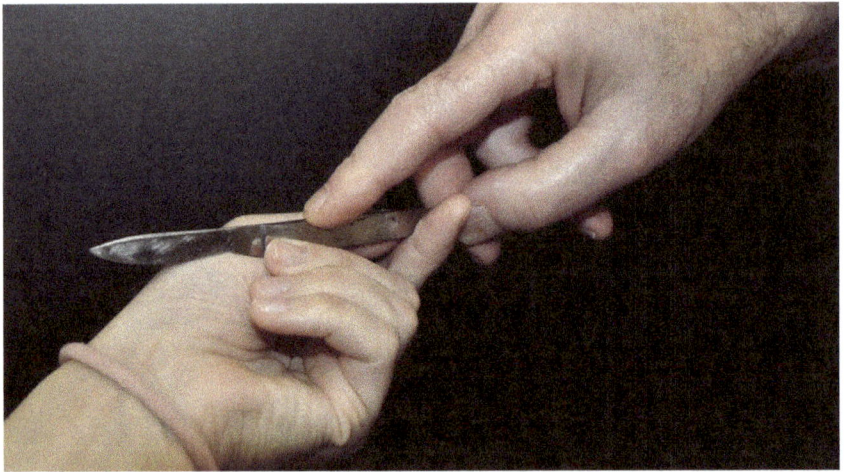

Figure 108.
Incorrect way to pass a knife to surgeon. Assistant's hand is on left. The assistant's hand should **never** be **under** the blade. The surgeon will grasp the handle and move it down which might cut into the assistant's palm. Knife-handles can also be transferred in kidney dishes

PASSING INSTRUMENTS

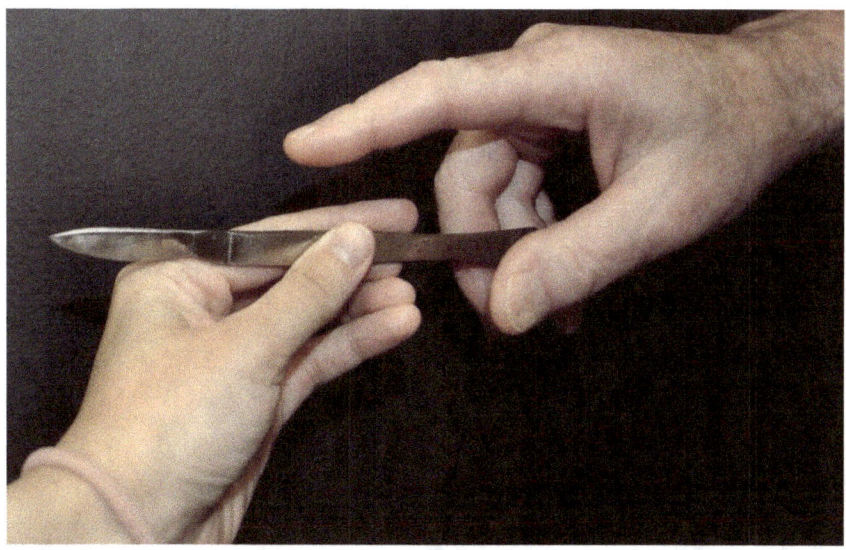

Figure 109.
Incorrect way to pass a knife to surgeon. Assistant's hand is on left. Assistant's hand should **never** be **under** the blade. The surgeon will grasp the handle and move it down thereby potentially cutting into the first web space of the assistant.

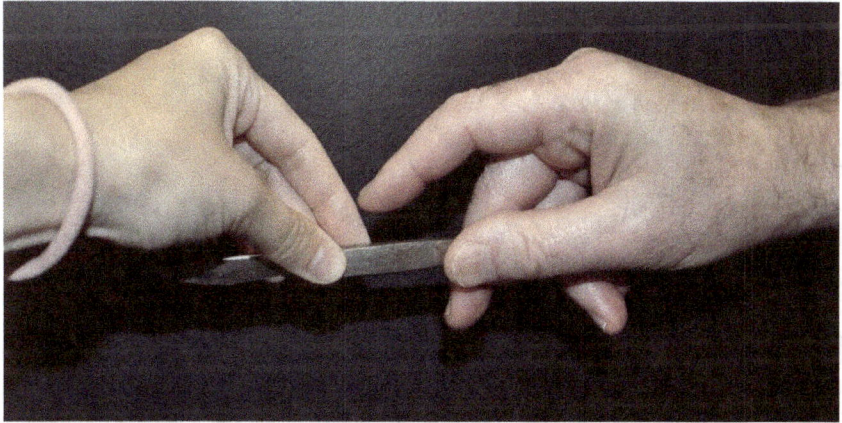

Figure 110.
Correct way to pass a knife. Assistant's hand is on left, surgeon's hand is on right. The blade is below the assistant's palm. There is no danger to the assistant as the surgeon receives the knife handle and brings his hand down,

C. Holding and passing a forceps

When passing a forceps place the handle firmly into the base of the first web space, between the thumb and index finger, with the toothed working-end pointing downwards.

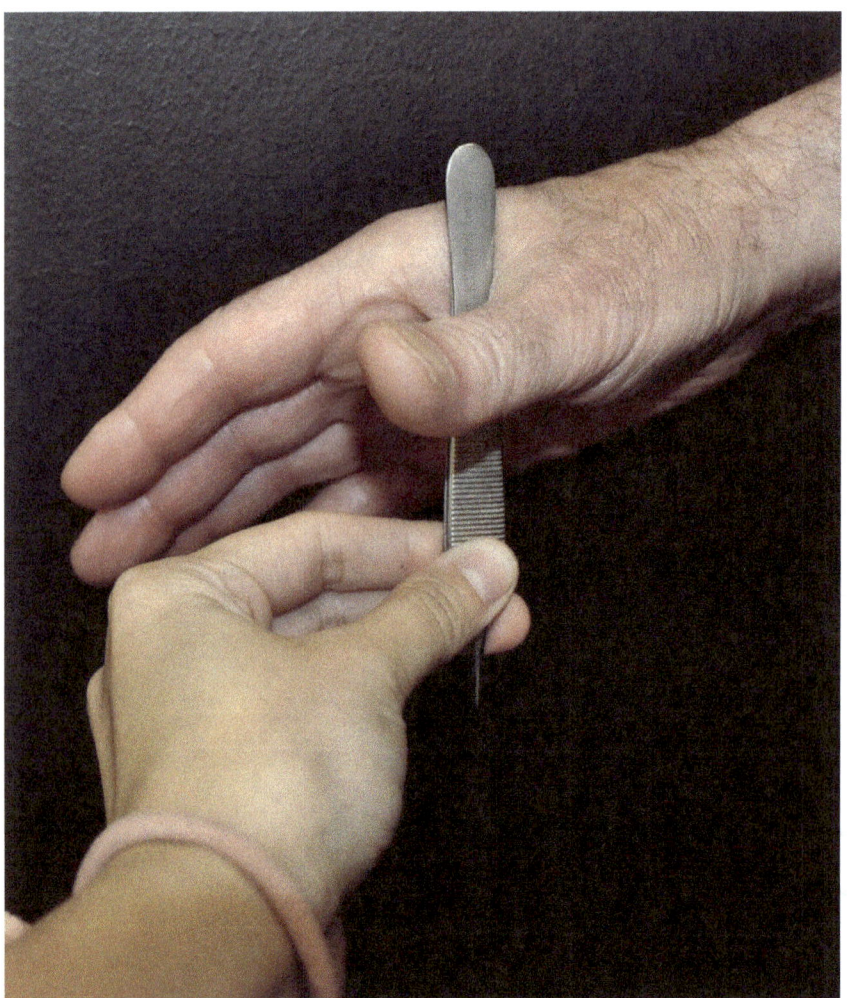

Figure 111
Passing forceps to the surgeon. Assistant's hand is on the left.

PASSING INSTRUMENTS

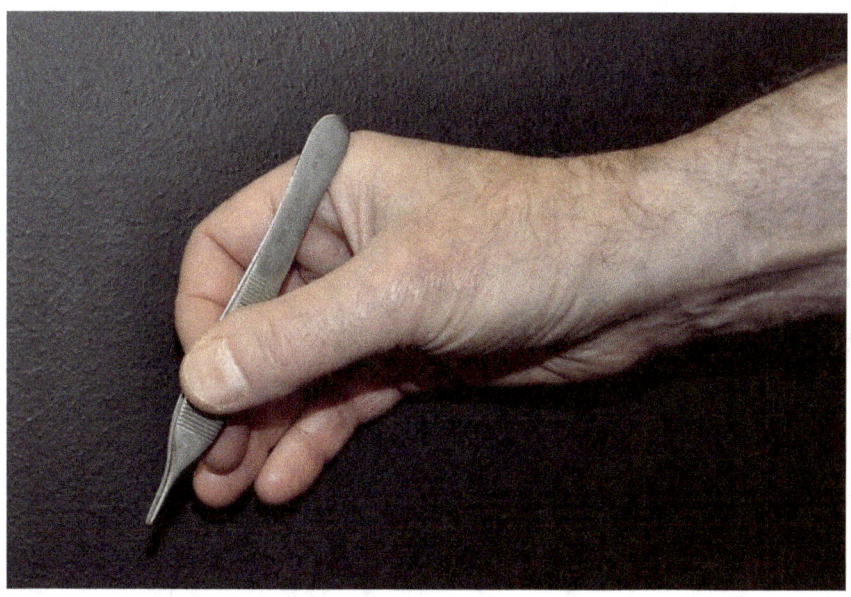

Figure 112.
Holding a forceps between the thumb and index.

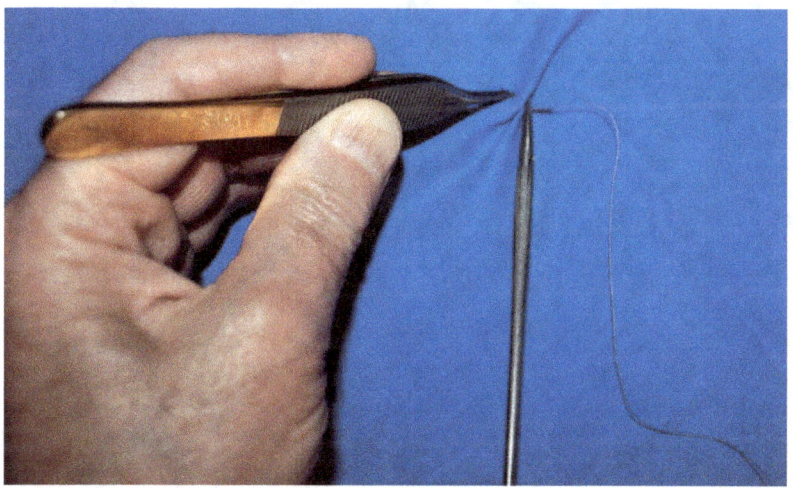

Figure 113.
A forceps is held firmly into the base of the first web space between the thumb and index finger, with the toothed end facing downward.

KIRWAN'S OPERATION ROOM TECHNIQUES

D. Passing a closed-handled instrument

An instrument with a handle such as a mallet, elevator, or a rasp should be placed with the handle in the palm.

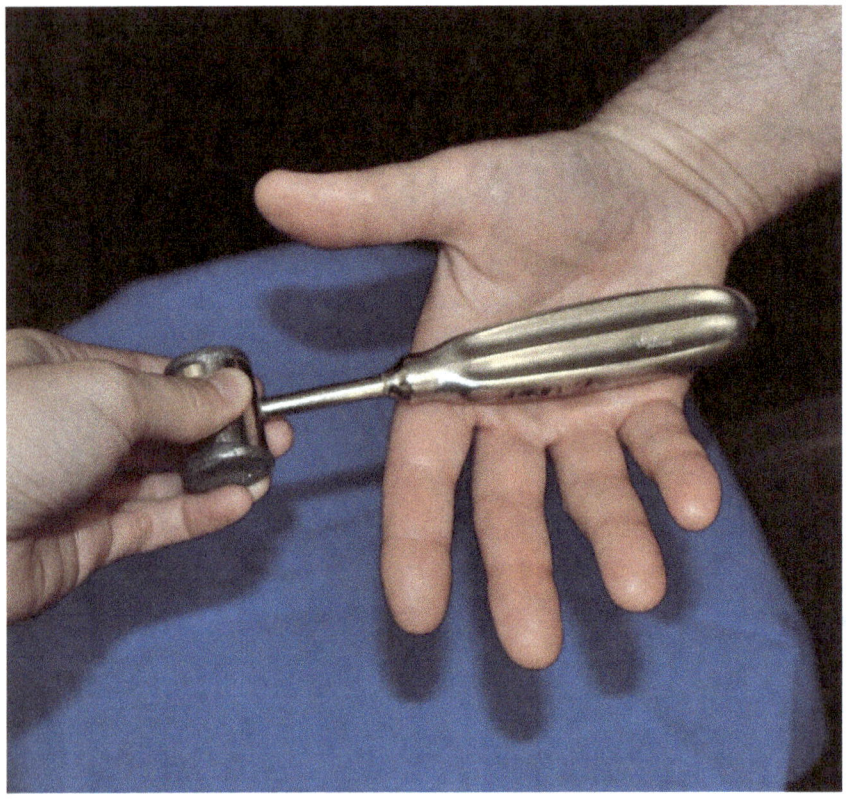

Figure 114.
Passing a mallet or instrument with a handle. A "handled" instrument such as a mallet, rasp, or elevator is placed in the surgeon's palm on the radial (thumb side) like a ring-handled instrument. Place the flat side of the handle in the palm, as shown.

PASSING INSTRUMENTS

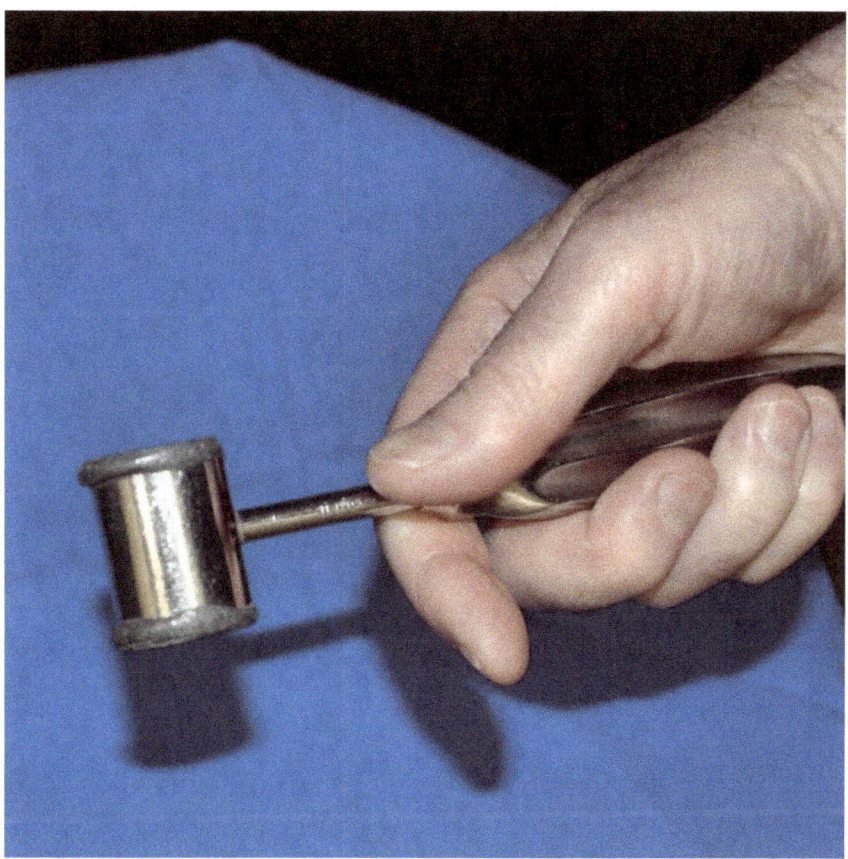

Figure 115.
Once in the surgeon's palm, the mallet can be grasped by closing the thumb and fingers around the handle as shown and can be used immediately. A rasp may be held in a similar fashion. An osteotome is held with the hand at the side so that the assistant can strike the end of the instrument with the mallet or hammer (not shown).

WOUND SPONGING

09

Open a Raytec sponge and hold it so that it is over your index finger.

Wipe the skin *surface* firmly with a sponge so that the surgeon can see the suture line. Remove the sponge so that the surgeon can place the next suture bite. When inside of a wound, Dab **firmly** and *do not wipe*.

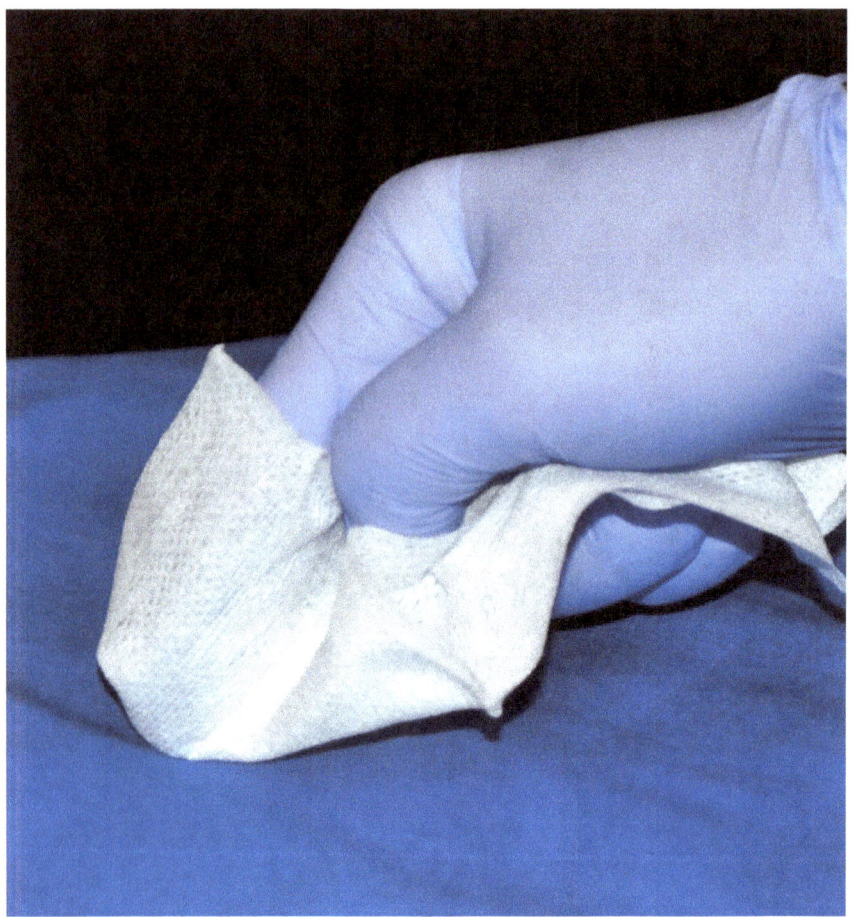

Figure 116.
Wound sponging with Raytec sponge over the index finger.

ERGONOMICS

10

Tips for maximum efficiency.

⟫ Do not allow your head or your hand to cross the line of vision between the surgeon's eye and the end of the surgeon's instrument. Imagine the surgeon is driving a car and you are the passenger. You would not want to put a hand in front of a driver's line of vision.

⟫ Always look at the operative field. Imagine you are the driver!

⟫ The operative field is a small area where the point of the surgeon's instrument is working.

⟫ Do not clean up blood or suture ends that are not in the operative field. It is distracting and does not help.

⟫ Sometimes, what you think may be a loose suture end may in fact be the end of the suture being placed. Pulling on it will pull on the needle holder and could pull the suture out and tear tissue! This happens surprisingly often and can be avoided.

⟫ Do not bend over, ever! Work at arm's length.

⟫ Alternatively, bend your knees or sit down. But keep your back straight.

⟫ If you need more light, move the overhead light. I If you can't reach it, ask for the circulator to bring it into your field.

⟫ If you are right-handed, position the overhead surgical light behind your right shoulder.

⟫ If you are left-handed, you should position the surgical light behind your left shoulder.

⟫ Release an instrument when the surgeon takes a hold of it in their hand. LET GO!!! It is not a tug-of-war!

⟫ Do not remove retractors or move other instruments until instructed to do so. If you think a retractor or other instrument is no longer needed, ask the surgeon if you can

ERGONOMICS

remove it. If you remove a retractor without asking, this may result in loss of exposure and may halt the procedure until the retractor is reinserted.

>>> Give each hand a task. Try not to let hands sit idle.

>>> Hold an instrument in the position it is given to you.

>>> *"Toe-in"* retractors so they do not slip out.

>>> If you cannot see to assist, say so. The surgeon needs your feedback to help you, so that you can help them.

>>> Attach a drain to its reservoir during the surgery, this saves time.

>>> Charge the reservoir when the wound is closed. See figures 117A and 117B.

>>> Do not push the bottom end of the bulb in. See Figure 118. This does not create suction. (See below). "In all sizes of drains, compressing the sides of the reservoir is a far better technique for establishing negative pressure than pressing the bottom of the drain up toward the top." *Carruthers, KH, et. al., Optimizing the Closed Suction Surgical Drainage System, Surgical Nursing, Jan–Mar 2013, Vol 33, No 1.*

>>> Squeeze the reservoir and push the stopper into the *correct* opening. Practice this outside the operating room. See figure 119.

>>> Secure the reservoir, with its clip, to the drapes so that it is not inadvertently pulled out during surgery or when the drapes are removed at the termination of the procedure.

>>> You get faster by eliminating unnecessary maneuvers. See correct technique in figures 30, 31, 32.

>>> It is better to work at a slower pace and do an excellent job that does not have to be redone.

KIRWAN'S OPERATION ROOM TECHNIQUES

>>> Speed comes with practice.

>>> It is important to learn to cut sutures reliably, at the correct length, *and* without hesitation. This will avoid frustrating the surgeon and prolonging operative time.

>>> Do not begin to cut a suture, only to change your mind to reposition your scissors for a different cut. One cut, every time.

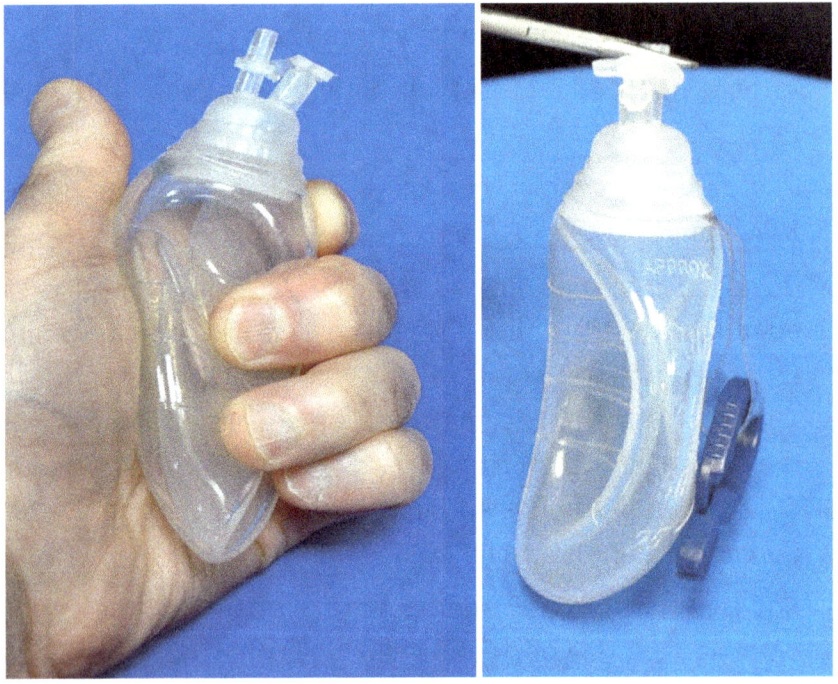

Figure 117A. and 117B.
Correct way to compress reservoir: negative pressure of 117.6 mmHg.

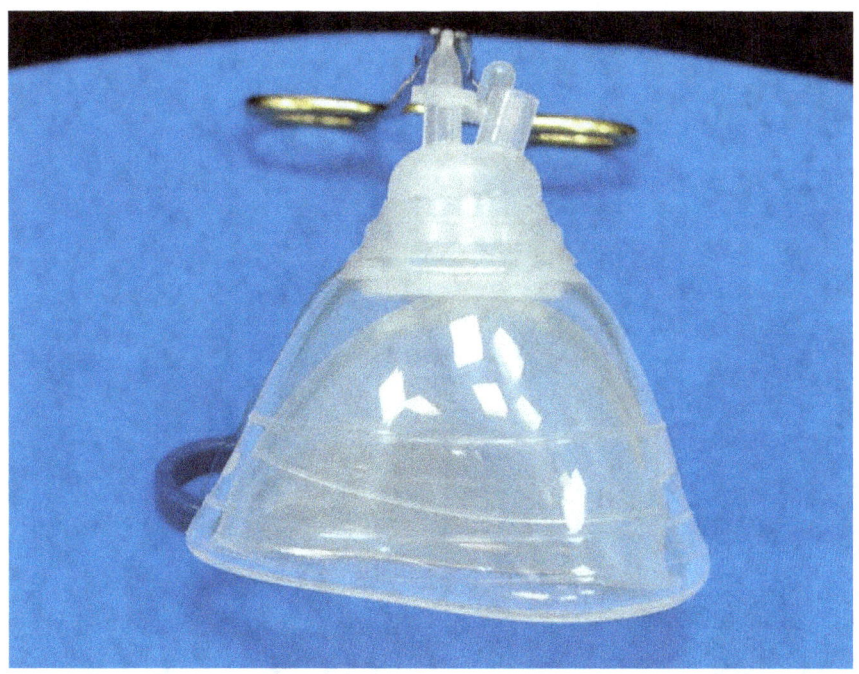

Figure 118.
Incorrect way to compress the drain reservoir: There is no measurable negative pressure.

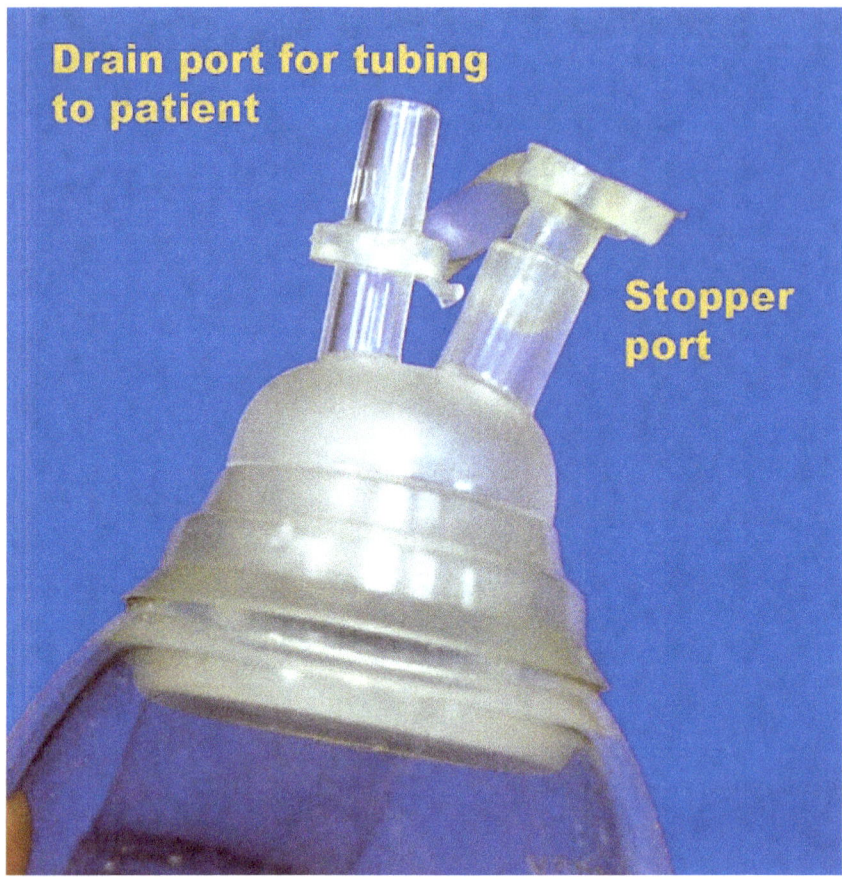

Figure 119.
Reservoir ports.

Use a two-handed surgeon's knot to secure a drain in so that you can cinch it down and compress the drain slightly, without it slipping. The drain should bulge slightly between the subsequent loops. The appearance should look like a "Roman Sandal." This is the most secure technique.

SAFETY

11

Safety tips

⟫ Always pass instruments and liquids **around** the face or the operative site.

⟫ Fluids must always be held **below the eye, nose, and ear canal.**

⟫ Touch instruments with the cautery at the instrument handle, not next to the skin. Touch the ring or the stem of the instrument to avoid the cautery tip inadvertently touching and burning the skin.

⟫ Use the side not the tip of the cautery blade, to touch the instrument, The tip of the blade gets covered with charred tissue debris, preventing a good electrical contact.

⟫ Use the blue button for cautery, not the yellow button. See Figure 120

⟫ Press on the cautery button until the surgeon says to stop, or until the surgeon releases the forceps or hemostat.

⟫ If the surgeon is constantly using the cautery, hold it in your hand and pass it to the surgeon each time she or he uses it, rather than placing it back into the holder (quiver) after each use.

⟫ Do not pass cords or suction tubing over the surgeon's left (non-dominant) forearm. If possible, pass them underneath the forearm so that the cord or tubing is kept out of the field and does not interfere with the surgeon's movements.

⟫ Do not lean or rest on the patient!

⟫ Do not leave a cautery tip resting on skin or drapes. Cautery tips are hot and can burn the skin and drapes even when they are not in use.

SAFETY

- ⟫ Metal instruments resting on the skin can cause burns when a grounded cautery is in use. Return instruments to the scrub nurse or place on a non-conductive pad.
- ⟫ Inadvertent stepping on a cautery pedal when the cautery tip is in contact with the skin or drapes can cause burns and fires.
- ⟫ Avoid leaving an active light cord on the drapes or the skin. The hot tip of the light cable can cause burns or fires. Turn the light source off when not in use.
- ⟫ Always hand instruments to the scrub nurse when not in use.
- ⟫ Keep the operative field tidy.
- ⟫ You can take instruments from the Mayo Stand if the scrub nurse approves.
- ⟫ If the surgeon asks for an instrument from the scrub, do not first take it from the scrub and then pass it to the surgeon. The surgeon should take the instrument directly from the scrub. To "relay" an instrument to the surgeon is time wasting and inefficient. Allow the scrub to place instruments directly into the surgeon's hand. However, there may be occasions when the scrub nurse is unable to reach the surgeon and will pass the instrument first to the assistant who then passes it to the surgeon.
- ⟫ Utilize your peripheral vision. Make sure that instruments, cautery units, suction tips, and suction tubing are safely secured and do not fall off the table. This is aggravating and creates unnecessary delays and expense to replace the lost item.

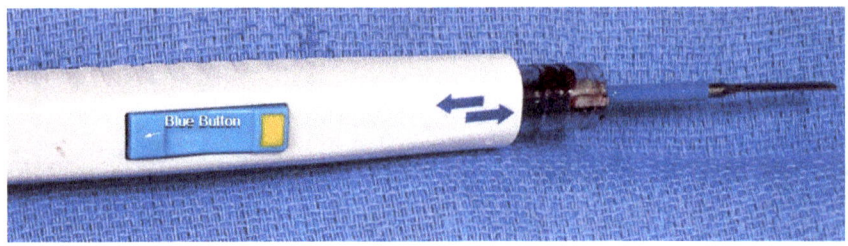

Figure 120.
The blue button is for coagulation.

ANTICIPATION

12

Always anticipate. Failure to anticipate is a common mistake but easily corrected. Anticipation is an easy skill to learn, and there is very little excuse for not mastering it at an early stage. Lack of anticipation gives an impression of inattention, lack of knowledge, or boredom.

Precipitating event	Response
Is the surgeon tying a suture?	Have scissors in your hand ready to cut it.
	Consider "palming" the scissors so they are ready to use when needed. .
Is there an actively bleeding vessel?	Grab a hemostat or a cautery or place your foot ready to depress the bipolar peddle.
Is there an actively bleeding vessel?	Have a Raytec sponge or laparotomy sponge at the ready.
Is there an actively bleeding vessel?	Alternatively, have suction ready to aspirate if asked. Be prepared!
Surgeon is using cautery repeatedly but intermittently for dissection or hemostasis	keep the cautery handle in your hand, ready to pass beck to the surgeon.

Table 8.
Tips for anticipation.

PRACTICE, PRACTICE, PRACTICE

13

Practice tips

>>> Carry a hemostat in your pocket so that you can learn how to hold it.

>>> Learn how the ratchet works. Practice releasing the ratchet mechanism with one hand, without looking.

>>> Practice two-handed knots, one-handed knots, and instrument ties.

>>> Practice surgeon's knots, square knots, and half-hitch knots.

>>> Do not just learn one-handed ties and instrument ties.

>>> Practice two-handed ties! This is a very important skill.

>>> Practice tightening down a half-hitch knot with the right index finger, keeping the other end taut.

>>> Practice tightening down a half-hitch knot using the left index,

>>> Practice outside the operating room. You will not achieve proficiency with these maneuvers and suture techniques if you only perform them during surgery. If you show an inability to perform these techniques, you will be given less to do in the OR because you will be too slow and show an obvious lack of practice.

>>> Be prepared.

>>> Read up on the scheduled surgical procedure and anatomy beforehand.

>>> Be early. Actors have a saying: "If you cannot be on time, be early!" Do not wait in the lounge for the surgeon. Be in the admissions area or, even better, in the operating room scrubbed, gowned, and ready to go

PRACTICE, PRACTICE, PRACTICE

>>> Don't be afraid to help as much as possible, be it helping to bring the patient into the OR, transferring them to the operating table, etc. The more you do, the more you will be given to do.

ABOUT THE AUTHOR

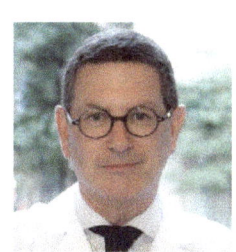

Laurence Kirwan was born in Liverpool, England. He graduated from the University of Manchester Medical School. He trained in Plastic Surgery at the University of Missouri, Kansas City. Dr. Kirwan has been in private practice in Plastic Surgery for over thirty-five years. He is a recognized national and international leader in Aesthetic Plastic Surgery of the face, breast, and body. Dr. Kirwan is certified by the American Board of Plastic Surgery and is a Fellow of the Royal College of Surgeon of England. In 1996, he was appointed Professor of Plastic Surgery at the International School of Aesthetic Plastic Surgery of the University of Belgrade. From 1996 until 2016, Dr. Kirwan trained other Plastic Surgeons in the Cosmetic Surgery Fellowship program at New York Eye & Ear Infirmary. He currently trains Physician Assistants within the Yale New Haven Health System Surgery Fellowship Program based at Norwalk Hospital. Dr. Kirwan has given over ten courses at the Annual Scientific Meetings of the American Society for Aesthetic Plastic Surgery (ASAPS) and the American Society of Plastic Surgeons (ASPS). He has also been invited as an expert panelist at many International Plastic Surgery meetings, and an invited Professor at the Siluetti Aesthetic Hospital in Helsinki, Finland.

His current hospital affiliations are Norwalk Hospital, Norwalk, and Greenwich Hospital, Greenwich, Connecticut. You can learn more about his practice and the procedures he performs at https://drkirwan.com. If you have any questions, please email him at info@drkirwan.com.

www.ingramcontent.com/pod-product-compliance
Lightning Source LLC
Chambersburg PA
CBHW050004230526
45465CB00003BB/1255